P9-DIG-208

THE PATIENT'S GUIDE TO PROSTATE CANCER

"This book provides you and your family members with the information you need to understand your disease and examine your treatment options. You are going to read about the optimal management of prostate cancer as far as we know it in the mid-1990s. You will also learn about promising new treatments that are now being investigated. You will get the facts, and you will also get the controversies, because your understanding of the issues can have enormous relevance for your getting the best possible medical care."
—Marc B. Garnick, M.D., from the Introduction

MARC B. GARNICK, M.D., is one of the country's leading experts on prostate cancer. A graduate of Bowdoin College and the University of Pennsylvania School of Medicine, he is a faculty member at Harvard Medical School, where he developed programs on the treatment of prostate cancer. He practices medicine at Boston's Beth Israel Hospital.

RC
280
.P7
G37
1996

THE PATIENT'S GUIDE TO PROSTATE CANCER

AN EXPERT'S SUCCESSFUL TREATMENT STRATEGIES AND OPTIONS

MARC B. GARNICK, M.D.

A PLUME BOOK

WITHDRAWN
KVCC
KALAMAZOO VALLEY
COMMUNITY COLLEGE
LIBRARY

MAR 8 1999

*To all my patients, from whom I have learned the most
about cancer, courage, hope, and healing, and
in particular to Horst J. Feist and the late Joseph Papp.*

PUBLISHER'S NOTE
The ideas, procedures, and suggestions contained in this book are not intended as a substitute for consulting with your physician. All matters regarding your health require medical supervision.

PLUME

Published by the Penguin Group
Penguin Books USA Inc., 375 Hudson Street, New York, New York 10014, U.S.A.
Penguin Books Ltd, 27 Wrights Lane, London W8 5TZ, England
Penguin Books Australia Ltd, Ringwood, Victoria, Australia
Penguin Books Canada Ltd, 10 Alcorn Avenue, Toronto, Ontario, Canada M4V 3B2
Penguin Books (N.Z.) Ltd, 182–190 Wairau Road, Auckland 10, New Zealand

Penguin Books Ltd, Registered Offices:
Harmondsworth, Middlesex, England

First published by Plume, an imprint of Dutton Signet,
a division of Penguin Books USA Inc.

First Printing, July, 1996
10 9 8 7 6 5 4 3

Copyright © Marc B. Garnick, 1996
All rights reserved

 REGISTERED TRADEMARK—MARCA REGISTRADA

LIBRARY OF CONGRESS CATALOGING-IN-PUBLICATION DATA:
Garnick, Marc B.
    The patient's guide to prostate cancer : an expert's successful treatment strategies and options / Marc B. Garnick.
        p.   cm.
    Includes bibliographical references and index.
    ISBN 0-452-27455-9
    1. Prostate—Cancer—Popular works.   I. Title.
RC280.P7G37   1996
616.99′463—dc20
                                                                        96-11170
                                                                        CIP

Printed in the United States of America
Set in New Baskerville
Designed by Jesse Cohen

Without limiting the rights under copyright reserved above, no part of this publication may be reproduced, stored in or introduced into a retrieval system, or transmitted, in any form, or by any means (electronic, mechanical, photocopying, recording, or otherwise), without the prior written permission of both the copyright owner and the above publisher of this book.

BOOKS ARE AVAILABLE AT QUANTITY DISCOUNTS WHEN USED TO PROMOTE PRODUCTS OR SER-VICES. FOR INFORMATION PLEASE WRITE TO PREMIUM MARKETING DIVISION, PENGUIN BOOKS USA INC., 375 HUDSON STREET, NEW YORK, NY 10014.

CONTENTS

ACKNOWLEDGMENTS

Over the past twenty years, I have been influenced by some extraordinary physicians involved in the care of patients with urologic cancer. It would be difficult to name them all, but many of these brilliant minds had tremendous influence in my development as a cancer specialist. During my medical school and house-staff training days at the University of Pennsylvania School of Medicine, I was fortunate to be a student of Dr. Samuel Thier, an individual of enormous talents who constantly instilled in me a desire to study as hard as I could, and know as much I could know. His command of the medical literature was unparalleled. Yet his caring for the patient as an individual was what impressed me most about Sam. It was this model of a learned, knowledgeable, but caring and compassionate physician that I have tried to follow.

My colleague Dr. Jerome Richie has been an important influence on my urologic cancer thinking. From 1982 to 1994, he and I have codirected a course on Urologic Cancer for the Department of Continuing Education at Harvard Medical School. Every two years, for an intensive three-day conference, we brought together the world's leading thinkers in the field of clinical urologic cancer research. Our course covered the most recent and emerging research concerning cancers of the kidney, bladder, testis, and of course the prostate gland. Physicians who particularly influenced me as a result of their teachings include Drs. Malcolm Bagshaw, George Canellos, Norman Coleman, J. Robert Cassady, William Catalona, William DeWolf, Lawrence Einhorn, William Fair, Emil Frei III, Gerald Hanks, Samuel Hellman, the late William Kaplan, Robert Mayer, Carl Olsen, Peter Scardino, William Shipley, Donald Skinner, Thomas Stamey, Patrick Walsh, the late Willet Whitmore, Jr., and the late Alan Yagoda. A course that disseminates the teaching of the great minds in prostate cancer will continue under my direction at the Beth Israel Hospital in Boston. I would also like to thank Dr. Miguel Srougi for sharing his experiences and the South American perspective with me. A special thanks also to Drs. David G. Nathan and Malcolm Gefter who have provided me with invaluable guidance and wisdom over the years.

Over the years, there have been a special few physicians I was fortunate enough to interact with, either as part of an individual clinical program, or in the clinical development of leuprolide. These include my special friends Dr. L. Michael Glode, Dr. Jay Smith, and Dr. Devorah Max. The exciting partnership that the four of us had in the development of leuprolide was a once-in-a-lifetime experience. I think we learned a great deal about prostate cancer during the course of those investigations.

A special thanks goes to Dr. William Fair, who has been kind enough to write a foreword to this book. Bill and I have spent countless hours together discussing the nuances of prostate cancer treatment—his from the perspective of a learned surgeon in charge of one of the largest cancer facilities in the world, and mine from that as a medical oncologist and someone with a keen interest in the drug development process as related to urologic cancer. These were collaborative problem-solving explorations in which the final outcome always seemed greater than the individual components. Bill, thanks so much for being there.

I could never have developed this book without the intimate involvement of my patients, who serve as the core of the book, as well as its inspiration. Dr. Thier always impressed upon me that if you listen to your patients, they will tell you exactly what is going on. He was 100 percent correct. Patients, if listened to carefully, will express things about their illness that you could never pick up in a textbook. I have learned and continue to learn something from each and every one of my patients. I know this will always continue as long as I am patient enough to continue to be a good listener. To my readers, I hope that you will get as much help, wisdom, and encouragement from reading about these patients as I have from knowing them.

To Robbie Butler, a close colleague and editorial assistant, a special and hearty thanks. A special thanks to Gabriel Schmergel and Ms. Tana Pesso, both of whom encouraged my professional development in many different ways. To Ricki Rusting, senior editor at *Scientific American*, I owe a great deal. By working on the *Scientific American* article which served as the foundation for this book, I learned a tremendous amount about translating scientific/medical information into a format for the lay public. Working with Ricki, many skills were developed that will hopefully make this book as intelligible and comprehensible as possible for the nonscientist and nonphysician. To my agent Ethan Ellenberg, a special thanks for working with me to make this manuscript as polished and as relevant as possible. To Carol Hart, I am indebted for her expert collaboration with me in putting the manuscript in its final form, with sensitive attention to both what readers needed to know and what I wished to express. I owe a great deal to Senior Editor Deborah Brody, and her unusually talented colleagues at Dutton.

Finally, I would like to thank my family for their unwavering support and loving encouragement—my parents Ruth and Philip Garnick, my two children Alex and Nathaniel, and my wife Bobbi Kates-Garnick, whose steadfast support, encouragement, advice, and wisdom helped shape this book from its inception.

FOREWORD

It is hardly possible to read the health sections of many newspapers or magazines without stumbling on an article about prostate cancer. The disease is now more prevalent than ever; nearly 250,000 new cases were diagnosed last year alone. But even though we are more aware of this disease, the man who has just been diagnosed may find it difficult to understand the nature of the illness and what the appropriate treatments for his condition are—indeed, the medical community continues to make new discoveries and to debate what approaches work best. In this exceptional book, Dr. Marc Garnick uses case histories gleaned from his twenty years of practice in caring for patients with prostate cancer to help readers make informed choices that meet their needs. Every man with prostate cancer, no matter how minimal or advanced his cancer is, will find invaluable information and in-depth discussion of his condition in this book. Additionally, men who are in the midst of being evaluated for possible prostate cancer will find crucial information here.

The issue of how to treat prostate cancer is complicated by the unpredictable nature of the disease and the paucity of definitive medical studies that examine the effectiveness of various treatments. One traditional view is that prostate cancer is a disease common to old age and is best left alone. Other doctors advocate more aggressive treatments, ranging from high-dose radiation to radical prostatectomy (surgery). A man just diagnosed with prostate cancer, and his family, will suddenly be called upon to determine what method of treatment is appropriate for him, perhaps turning to the many articles and books about the disease for information and guidance. While many of these publications overwhelm the reader with medical jargon and statistics, Dr. Garnick, who is on the leading edge of prostate cancer treatment and research, has written a book that is clear, concise, and up-to-date. He guides readers through the maze of often conflicting information about how to diagnose and treat prostate cancer in an authoritative yet accessible tone. When no clear-cut conclusions can be reached from the available clinical research, Dr. Garnick articulates his own approaches to management and treatment thoughtfully and intelligently, and supports his conclusions with his considerable experience in treating prostate cancer patients.

I have been fortunate enough to work with Dr. Garnick many times. His knowledge of prostate cancer is encyclopedic, and he is a compassionate physician and a first-rate scientist and researcher who fully understands the issues involved in prostate cancer care; readers who have just found out they have prostate cancer could not be in better hands. He discusses in detail every diagnostic procedure, explores all possible treatments and approaches, from the conventional to the controversial, and offers invaluable advice in how men can improve the quality and quantity of their lives after their diagnosis.

Our understanding of prostate cancer is rapidly changing, and now more than ever it is vital that patients have reliable resources they can go to for information and support. Dr. Garnick is a pioneer in the field of prostate cancer research and treatment who has helped countless men battle the disease. This book will become a standard reference for patients with prostate cancer and their families.

—William R. Fair, M.D.
Memorial Sloan Kettering Cancer Institute
New York, New York

INTRODUCTION

The news that you have—or might have—prostate cancer is hard to take. Your immediate reaction may be disbelief, anger, fear, denial, a feeling of helplessness, or all of the above. This book is written to help you cope with any confusion you may be feeling right now, and to guide you through the whole process of diagnosing, treating, and monitoring prostate cancer, whether early or advanced.

This book provides you and your family members with the information you need to understand your disease and examine your treatment options. You are going to read about the optimal management of prostate cancer as far as we know it in the midnineties. You will also learn about promising new treatments that are now being investigated. You will get the facts, and you will also get the controversies, because your understanding of the issues can have enormous relevance for your getting the best possible medical care.

Our ability to detect and treat prostate cancer has expanded enormously over the past decade. If, like most newly diagnosed prostate cancer patients, your disease was detected on a screening test before you had any symptoms, your cancer is probably still small and confined to your prostate. This means you have an excellent chance of a total cure. However, we don't yet know the long-term outcome of our new, expanded ability to detect and treat. We haven't accumulated enough hindsight to know what is the most appropriate treatment for each type of prostate cancer.

Both the disease itself and the treatments for it can cause urinary and sexual complications. Some treatments with fewer side effects have a higher risk of cancer recurrence. Some prostate cancers spread rapidly, others cause no symptoms for years. Evaluating the options and balancing the trade-offs can be very difficult. It should be done by you and your family in conjunction with your doctor, not by either one of you alone.

You, the patient, have to make the final decision regarding treatment. One prominent physician caring for women with breast cancer makes this point. The physician, he says, is an expert on the medical aspects of the disease and the treatment. The patient is the expert on how he (or she) wants to live his (or her) life. You must try to be fully informed about the choices, expected results, and possible side effects, along with the overall impact that your cancer and treatment will have on your life.

If you are confused or overwhelmed, read slowly, in stages. An index and a glossary are provided to help you find your way. Some sections may go into greater depth than what you need to know right now. If you have been diagnosed with early-stage cancer with no evidence of spread, for example, there is no reason for you to read about the management of advanced, treatment-resistant disease.

As you read, I suggest that you pay attention to your feelings and reactions. Are you tending to focus on the worst-case scenario or the best-case scenario, to the exclusion of all the other possibilities? Does one possibility seem so overwhelmingly terrible that you would do anything to avoid it? Realize that there are some very tolerable ways of managing prostate cancer and going on with life. You will read about a few patients who did not get adequate treatment or who had unexpected complications. Don't allow these stories to make you feel either helpless or hopeless. By learning about prostate cancer, by reading this book, you take a big step toward minimizing your chance of a bad outcome.

Trust your doctor, listen to your doctor, but realize that he or she does not know everything. Your doctor can be extremely competent and caring, yet still make a decision that does not go well. To minimize that possibility, you need to learn as much as possible about prostate cancer, so that you can be an active, well-informed partner in deciding your own treatment.

Fear of cancer, fear of the complications of treatment, can lead patients to make poor or irrational decisions. One focused on the good news, asked no questions, and did not return for follow-up. Another never stopped asked questions—putting treatment off indefinitely as he read medical journals and interviewed all the experts. Two of the patients you will read about wanted every possible treatment, no matter how severe the side effects or how limited the benefits. Other patients found the possibility of incontinence or impotence unacceptable, and chose treatments that had a greater risk of cancer recurrence. Again, only you can know your quality-of-life requirements. But be sure you really know them. Let your cancer-treatment decision be the most carefully considered and best-informed decision of your life.

In my experience, answers to their questions are what patients want most. This book combines the most current medical information and medical judgment with true case histories, so that you will be able to use the experiences of others to evaluate your own situation. If you, the reader, feel that you have gained insight into prostate cancer treatment through reading about these patients and my decision-making discussions with them, then my vision of this book will be achieved.

PATIENT PROFILES

In the pages that follow, you will be introduced to a few of the many remarkable patients I have had the privilege to know in over twenty-five years of practicing medicine. None are likely to be exactly like you, either in terms of medical condition, life history, personal situation, or preferences for treatment. Yet, as you read on and learn more about them, their stories may help you understand your own circumstances and the options before you a little better.

For the sake of confidentiality, in all but one instance their names and other identifying details have been changed.

If some details in these introductory sketches are unclear to you, reading on or checking the glossary may help. A PSA (prostate-specific antigen) blood test is used to detect and monitor prostate problems. The higher the level, or the more rapidly the level rises over time, the greater the chance of significant cancer. The PSA level should drop to zero after prostate surgery if the cancer was confined to the prostate. In addition to the PSA blood test, the other important test to detect prostate problems is the digital rectal examination, or DRE. With this test the physician places a finger in the rectum and is able to feel and evaluate the prostate gland.

*   *   *

Ted Kazarian, a sixty-nine-year-old professional, had his PSA level double from 4.5 to 9.1 ng/ml in one year. (A reading under 4.0 is generally considered normal, and rapidly increasing levels suggest cancer.) Two separate sets of biopsies of the prostate gland were performed, both of which were negative. Mr. Kazarian will need to have regular PSA tests to monitor his level, but when two separate sets of biopsies show no signs of cancer, the odds are very much in his favor that he is cancer-free. And even if cancer is present, it is likely to be insignificant cancer.

Alfred Owens, a seventy-year-old retired technician, was told that his prostate cancer was incurable and that treatment with hormones would be the least invasive and most tolerable choice. He resigned himself to a brief period of cancer remission, followed by metastatic disease and death. The hormonal treatment did shrink his cancer, and when he came to see me, I recommended that we "go for a cure" by adding radiation treatment. The idea that a cure might be possible brought Mr. Owens out of his depression and hopelessness. Nearly two years later, all evidence of cancer is gone, and his PSA value is now 0 ng/ml.

Douglas Fiedler, a sixty-two-year-old educator, had an elevated PSA in the 10–12 ng/ml range, as well as a long-standing history of prostate infection, which can raise the PSA level. One set of eight needle biopsies was negative for cancer. When the PSA remained high after antibiotic treatment of the infection, another set of eight biopsies was performed. One biopsy showed cancer. Many different opinions were offered about the best treatment approach before it was decided to remove the prostate (radical prostatectomy). Mr. Fiedler developed a severe and unusual type of bowel infection after surgery that delayed his recovery. Today he is well.

Viktor Gabler, a sixty-one-year-old European businessman, delayed treatment for two years, perhaps because European physicians often opt not to treat prostate cancer. Mr. Gabler's father had died of prostate cancer. When evaluated at our center, Mr. Gabler had a slightly elevated PSA of 7.6 ng/ml, a biopsy positive for cancer, and an abnormal area on bone scan, suggesting the possibility that the prostate cancer had spread to the bone. Again, his doctors had different opinions about the next diagnostic or treatment step. The PSA value and the type of cancer found in the biopsy strongly suggested his disease was still localized to the prostate, and Mr. Gabler was spared having to undergo a biopsy of the abnormal bone.

George Parisi, a seventy-three-year-old consultant, had an initial PSA value of 7.1 ng/ml, which had increased to 7.4 one year later. A prostate biopsy showed cancer, but the lymph-node biopsy was negative, indicating that the cancer was localized. Many physicians would opt not to treat such a patient, assuming that he was more likely to die with, rather than of, his disease. Mr. Parisi and I made the decision to treat, since he was otherwise healthy and active. He underwent a radical prostatectomy and today is doing well, with a PSA of zero.

Wilson Orr, a vigorous and athletic sixty-five-year-old, was told he had metastatic cancer when the results of a PSA screening test showed a level of 200 ng/ml and the prostate biopsy revealed cancer. The diagnosis of metastatic cancer was based only on the PSA level. He was given hormone therapy and otherwise brushed aside as incurable. Six months into his treatment, a visit to our center raised the possibility that his cancer might be localized and curable. Mr. Orr is now doing well, tolerating radiation treatments without problems, and has a PSA below 2 ng/ml.

Kevin Loftus, a fifty-two-year-old university administrator, had a PSA level that kept doubling every year for four years, but was still in what is considered the normal range. Then his PSA level rose from 4 to 8 ng/ml, but six months went by before further tests were done, demonstrating cancer. He underwent surgery, but the cancer was too extensive to be operable. Much can still be done to control Mr. Loftus' cancer and prolong his survival in meaningful ways, but he may be one of the unfortunate ones who eventually die of their disease.

Daniel Husik, a sixty-eight-year-old teacher, was diagnosed with prostate cancer after a routine physical and PSA screening test. He had his prostate removed and his PSA dropped to zero. But the pathology report on his prostate showed a positive margin—meaning some cancer cells were still in the body. Five years later, his PSA level was creeping upward, though still quite low. At his request, he was given radiation treatments, which he tolerated very well.

Melvin Parks, a seventy-two-year-old retired factory worker, underwent radiation treatment for apparently localized cancer. His PSA before radiation treatment was 15 ng/ml and never dropped to zero. Now, four years after completion of his radiation treatments, Mr. Parks's PSA is in the 8–10 ng/ml range. He is very concerned and wants something done to bring the value back down. However, the best approach to cases such as his is not clear. Should the physician continue to monitor until there are more clear signs of disease, or undertake another round of treatment on the basis of a blood test?

Alan Quint was diagnosed with metastatic prostate cancer at the age of fifty-four. His cancer was successfully controlled with hormonal therapy for a time, but eventually became resistant to treatment. Over the later course of his illness, there were problems with family and significant others as Mr. Quint dealt with his fear of death, his self-pity, and his unwillingness to burden others. The family was very much involved in group discussions about whether it was better to attempt to extend Mr. Quint's survival time through experimental treatments, or to focus on keeping him at home and comfortable for the time left to him.

Donald Young, a seventy-five-year-old Ph.D. still active in his field, developed metastatic prostate cancer within one year after radiation treatment for apparently localized cancer. He had been treated with several hormonal drugs but his cancer was now resistant (refractory) to his treatment. Yet he was pain-free and without symptoms. He and his family insisted on further treatment, even though the few options left would only diminish his quality of life with very little or no benefit. I recognized the patient and family's right to make such a decision, but I still felt further treatment was not in Dr. Young's interest, and reluctantly withdrew from participating in his treatment.

Walter Kane, a fifty-eight-year-old producer with metastatic disease, wanted everything possible done to eliminate his cancer. He was treated with a number of experimental and standard treatments, including chemotherapy, hormonal therapy, and localized radiation therapy. Now, nine years later, he is cancer-free, but at a great cost in terms of quality of life. He is impotent and feels inadequate in his relationship with his wife. He has urinary problems that prevent him from working in his field. Mr. Kane never questions the value of being alive and disease-free this many years, but the "price of cure" has been quite significant.

John Konrad, a sixty-two-year-old engineer with international recognition in his field, sought medical attention for urinary and sexual symptoms. His physical exam and his PSA level suggested the possibility of cancer, so a biopsy was made. The "fine print" in the pathologist's report definitely suggested cancer, but Mr. Konrad's physician apparently did not read the report thoroughly and did not speak with the pathologist. He told Mr. Konrad to return for a reevaluation in six months. Falsely reassured and very busy, Mr. Konrad did not return for a year and a half, when his symptoms were much more severe. At this point he had advanced metastatic cancer. He is receiving hormonal therapy, but there is no expectation of a cure.

Martin Gorman, fifty years old, had localized prostate cancer. Because his sexual ability was very important to him, he opted for a type of prostate surgery that is designed to spare the nerves needed for an erection. Unfortunately, he did not recover his potency after the operation. He was able to achieve an erection using injections, but he disliked the process and became discouraged and depressed. When he came to see me again, I referred him to another specialist. Somehow, the "chemistry" between the two of them worked, and Mr. Gorman didn't find the injections so objectionable.

Jack Wilkins, sixty-two years old with early prostate cancer, claimed to be impotent with his wife but was involved in a long-term extramarital relationship. His wife could not understand why her husband wanted the nerve-sparing operation, since there is an increased risk that some of the cancer will be missed. He was able to continue his sexual activities on a somewhat reduced level afterward, but his PSA eventually started to rise. He is now undergoing radiation treatment.

Stephen Fisher, sixty-six years old, was also having an extramarital affair but was unable to perform sexually with his wife. Although she felt he would be best treated with surgery, Mr. Fisher opted for radiation. He is doing well and has maintained his sexual activity following completion of the radiation therapy.

Robert Bendler, a fifty-three-year-old banker, has had a PSA in the 10–12 ng/ml range for a number of years. A first biopsy found only benign enlargement and infection. A later biopsy showed cancer. He has received very different opinions regarding treatment and came to me for an additional evaluation. He chose a nonnerve-sparing surgery, along with an implant in the penis that allows him to have an erection and perform sexually.

James Rainey, an active fifty-three-year-old contractor, had an elevated PSA that was rising rapidly. A biopsy showed a type of cancer that often spreads aggressively. After much discussion, he opted for a series of hormonal therapies, to be followed by either radiation therapy or surgery. After the hormonal therapies, his PSA dropped to less than 0.5 ng/ml. He will have a nerve-sparing prostate surgery in the hope of curing his cancer without loss of sexual potency.

Michael Malloy, a forty-nine-year-old sales representative, had a family history of prostate cancer and had developed sexual problems. At the urging of his wife, he was screened for PSA level, which was 6.5 ng/ml. His biopsy, like Mr. Rainey's, showed an aggressive type of cancer, and he chose a similar series of treatment. Because the treatment was not recognized as a "standard option" by his health-insurance company, much correspondence and persuasion were needed before his treatment was approved for coverage.

Samuel Taggert, sixty-two years old with advanced emphysema, was diagnosed with prostate cancer after a PSA screening. Since he was ill already, it was not clear how he should be treated, or whether he should be treated at all. Surgery was extremely risky because of his lung disease. Mr. Taggert chose to receive radiation treatments at a hospital near his winter home in the South. He developed a complication of radiation therapy that, along with his lung disease, left him very ill and eventually bedridden until his death from emphysema three years after diagnosis with prostate cancer. Complications happen, and the hospital and staff may well be blameless, but his story points to the need to read and ask questions before you select both your treatment and the physicians who will be providing it.

Charles Becker, a highly successful, hard-driving businessman, was sixty years old when he was diagnosed with prostate cancer. After his initial shock, he threw all his energies into finding out everything he could, reading the medical literature and talking to all the experts. When he came to see me, I felt he wanted to display his own learning rather than hear my opinions about his treatment options. Over a year after his diagnosis, he has yet to be treated—because there is always another doctor to be consulted, another new study or research report to be considered.

Joseph Papp, Director of the New York State Shakespeare Festival and Public Theater: The story of Mr. Papp's battle with prostate cancer was well known at the time and is told in his biography, published after his death. He was sixty-five years old when he was diagnosed with prostate cancer in 1987. His PSA was nearly 200 ng/ml and a bone scan revealed extensive metastatic cancer, yet he was almost symptom-free. He had an extraordinary response to treatment that kept the cancer in complete remission for four very full and creative years.

The courage, vitality, and frankness of men like Mr. Papp help to educate others about the epidemic of prostate cancer and the possibility of living fully in its presence—to go for a cure if a cure is possible, or to select a treatment that will give you as many months or years of full, meaningful life as possible.

1

WHAT DOES IT MEAN TO HAVE PROSTATE CANCER?

It has long been taught in medical school that prostate cancer is an "old man's disease"—a very common and slow-growing type of cancer that rarely causes death. It has been estimated that nearly ten million men over age forty-five have small, undetectable prostate cancers. Such staggering numbers come from studies in which men die from other causes, and at the time of autopsy, the prostate gland is found to contain small areas of cancer. It has also been taught that prostate cancer is a disease that men die *with*, rather than *of*. Witness, for example, all the many men with prostate cancer who don't know they have it.

The other argument that prostate cancer is an old man's cancer and is best left alone relates to the finding of microscopic cancer in the prostate tissue of men treated for benign (noncancerous) prostate-gland enlargement (benign prostatic hyperplasia or BPH). This common condition of aging is often treated by surgically removing "chips" of the gland to relieve urinary difficulties caused by the gland's enlargement. When the tissue chips are examined under the microscope, small areas of cancer are sometimes found. Often this cancer does not require additional treatment, further supporting the traditional view that prostate cancer, if diagnosed, needs no active treatment intervention.

These common attitudes about prostate cancer need to be reexamined in light of the increased incidence of the disease currently affecting many younger men. There has never been a time in modern medical history in which the incidence of a cancer has soared as rapidly as prostate cancer. In 1996, there will be nearly 318,000 newly diagnosed cases, and the patients will tend to be much younger men than those diagnosed five or ten years earlier. This extaordinary number of newly diagnosed cases makes prostate cancer the most common cancer in males, and the second leading cause of cancer death among men. With widespread use of the PSA screening test, which can diagnose very early phases of the disease, it is likely that the number of reported cases will continue to rise at unprecedented rates.

Now that we have "found" all these once undetectable cases of early prostate cancer, what will we do with them? Many physicians still prescribe only "watchful waiting" for these early, often microscopic cancers in the belief that most prostate cancers are slow growing. However, if and when such a cancer does advance to cause symptoms, it is much more difficult to treat and a cure may not be possible.

There certainly are patients diagnosed with prostate cancer who are best managed with a "watchful waiting" policy. A perfect example would be a man in his eighties or nineties who is found to have prostate cancer but also suffers from other acute or chronic medical conditions, some of which may be life threatening. Since there are risks and complications involved in treating prostate cancer, these patients may have very little to gain, and much to lose, from being treated.

For younger or healthier men, there are risks in delaying treatment. Some patients who are found to have microscopic cancer that is believed to be "latent" or "indolent" later develop advanced, life-threatening forms of prostate cancer. A latent or indolent cancer is one that grows slowly, causes no symptoms, and is unlikely to spread throughout the body (metastasize). These are the cancers one is more likely to "die with" than "die of." Latent cancers are in direct contrast to aggressive or "virulent" cancers which, when identified and diagnosed, usually demand active treatment. There are approaches for trying to identify which cancers are latent and which are likely to be aggressive, but these evaluations are only predictions of the most likely course of the disease, and they are not always right.

In my view, the traditional teaching that prostate cancer is a disease men "die with" rather than "die of" is out of date medically and culturally. Our available treatments for prostate cancer are rapidly improving, despite the low level of research funding for this disease. We are generally living longer and more active lives than our grandparents did, and we are discovering that many of the conditions we once considered natural and inevitable aging processes, such as BPH in men and osteoporosis in women, are in fact diseases that can be treated or controlled. I regularly recommend treatment for active, otherwise healthy prostate cancer patients in their seventies and beyond. A healthy seventy-five-year-old man today has a life expectancy of about nine years, and a healthy man of eighty can expect to live seven more years. Shouldn't those seven to nine years be as disease-free as we have the capability to make them? For men diagnosed at an early age and in an early stage of the cancer, I believe there are even more compelling reasons to treat rather than wait and see if the cancer advances.

I have made every honest attempt to provide the most current and objective information available, but I also want you to know where I stand on the not-so-objective issues of when to treat and how to treat. I come to this topic as a medical oncologist, a physician whose primary role is treating patients with advanced, metastatic cancer—cancer which is no longer curable. In my view, there are diagnostic and treatment procedures now on the horizon that can substantially change the natural history or course of prostate cancer. Whenever I see a patient with incurable disease, I ask whether that patient, if diagnosed earlier and treated aggressively, could have been cured of his prostate cancer, and avoided the fate of dying from metastatic prostate cancer—a fate suffered by nearly forty-one thousand men in 1995.

You need to be aware that there are a number of controversies in prostate cancer medicine. The specialists and the experts do not agree on when to treat and how to treat. This does not mean that some are right and some are wrong, or that you are necessarily in danger of getting bad advice. Rather, it simply means that all the facts are not yet in. Because of the range of opinions and options available, I believe it is vitally important for you and your family to understand as much as possible about how medical decisions are made in the diagnosis and treatment of prostate cancer.

After physicians review the findings of the clinical examination and the diagnostic tests, they give their recommendation for treatment—which is of course known as an "opinion." Never forget the ordinary meaning of that ordinary word. Specialists are trained and experienced in selecting the patients for whom they can do the most good with the lowest risk of complications. However, surgeons are naturally inclined to recommend surgery, while radiation therapists are more likely to support the use of their mode of treatment. In some situations, the most appropriate treatment option is readily decided after discussions involving the patient, the family, and the physicians consulted. In other cases, there can be many different opinions about the extent of the cancer, and how—or whether—it should be treated.

For example, one patient you will read about, Douglas Fiedler, a sixty-two-year-old, otherwise healthy man, was first diagnosed with prostate infection (prostatitis), then later had two series of eight prostate biopsies. Because of the associated prostatitis, it was difficult to interpret his biopsies, which were reviewed by a total of four pathologists before a diagnosis of cancer was agreed upon. Then Mr. Fiedler's physicians disagreed on the appropriate treatment. His urologist felt the cancer found was of little significance. A radiation therapist believed that treatment was necessary, but did not want to treat with radiation therapy for fear that it would make the prostatitis worse. A second radiation therapist thought that radiation treatments were appropriate and was willing to treat the patient. Two medical oncologists (cancer specialists) thought that treatment was necessary, and it was the patient's choice to select between radiation and surgery (a radical prostatectomy, to remove the entire prostate gland). A second urologist and a third medical oncologist (myself) recommended treatment with radical prostatectomy.

Mr. Fiedler opted for the surgery. When the prostate was biopsied after surgery it did show several small areas of cancer. However, a severe bacterial infection occurred after surgery, prolonging Mr. Fiedler's hospitalization. Today he is well and considered cured.

His case is unusual, though not unique, in the number of specialists involved—two urologists, four pathologists, three medical oncologists, and two radiation therapists—who had differing views of the appropriateness or the necessity for treatment. The point which deserves emphasis here is that no one was right or wrong. Rather, there were several treatment choices and the one that was selected made sense to the patient, his family, and the treating physicians. Those who recommended treatment discharged their responsibilities and obligations by, hopefully, curing him, while those who argued for watchful waiting still believe that this particular cancer did not need treatment. We do not yet know the natural course of the type of tumor Mr. Fiedler had. I generally recommend treatment, as I did in this case, hoping to prevent the development of metastatic disease ten to fifteen years later. Although his case was difficult to diagnose and he experienced an unexpected complication, Mr. Fiedler was fortunate that he did receive good, well-considered medical advice, along with the information he needed to make his own decision.

Some patients are not so fortunate. In John Konrad's case, which you will also read more about, the initial pathologist's report on his biopsy suggested that there might be cancer present without providing a definite diagnosis. It would have been appropriate for the pathologist and the physician to discuss the report, and then perhaps consult another pathologist with more experience in this area. Apparently, there was no direct communication between the pathologist and the physician about the biopsy. Dr. Konrad's physician read the report hastily and did not pick up on the suspicious details of the biopsy. He told Dr. Konrad the biopsy was negative and to come back in six months for follow-up. Although Dr. Konrad had many symptoms that had not been explained or resolved, he took the happy news that he was cancer-free at face value. He did not return for follow-up for a year and a half. At this point, his prostate cancer was quite advanced and had metastasized to other parts of the body.

You should not conclude from the stories of Douglas Fiedler and John Konrad that you need multiple consults (second, third, fourth, fifth, and sixth opinions) in order to receive adequate diagnosis and treatment. On the contrary, I have occasionally encountered patients whose excessive "doctor shopping" needlessly postponed necessary treatment. Of these, Charles Becker was by far the most memorable.

When he was diagnosed with prostate cancer, Mr. Becker used his considerable wealth to gain as much information about his disease as possible. He or his staff did literature searches at medical libraries and identified the most prominent physicians and institutions for interpreting his biopsy slides, providing radiation treatment, or doing prostate surgery with low rates of complications. He sent his prostate biopsy slides to at least five separate institutions for interpretation. He sought consultations with at least four urologic cancer surgeons, two radiation oncologists, and had conversations with at least two pathologists. The process of getting this multitude of consultations took at least four months, during which Mr. Becker had still not decided on treatment.

Mr. Becker saw me following publication of my article, "The Dilemmas of Prostate Cancer," in *Scientific American.* When I met him, I was struck by his greater interest in holding an academic debate rather than entering into a physician-patient relationship. It was as though we were panel members in an international symposium debating all the controversial aspects of prostate cancer, where no one possessed truth, but people articulated their views, based on experience and beliefs about the disease.

When he posed a question and I provided an answer, he would counter with literature citations and notes that he had taken during his various interviews with others, trying to get me into a "gotcha" situation. During our meeting, I brought up the possibility of an investigational (not yet standard) treatment you will read about in a later chapter, called neoadjuvant hormonal therapy. He had not yet heard about this therapy, so it took some explaining before he understood it. As weird as it sounds, I felt he was more annoyed at himself for not having known about neoadjuvant hormonal therapy than interested in the possible benefit it might have for treating his individual cancer!

Patients have a right to know and to question. Let us not forget the case of Dr. Konrad, where asking more questions and demanding more information might have led to having his pathology report reviewed and studied more thoroughly.

While I admire and encourage a patient who wants to know as much as possible about his disease, I felt unfulfilled in my role as a consulting physician in trying to provide advice and counsel to Mr. Becker. After all, he had not made an appointment as an individual doing a research project on prostate cancer, but instead came to me as a patient with a malignant condition who needed some medical advice and judgment. I attempted during both the consult visit and in later telephone conversations to get this point across, but he only wanted to increase his information base about prostate cancer.

Not all patients, unfortunately, have equal access to the best available medical care. Geography, income, and restrictions imposed by insurers can all create barriers. African-Americans have the highest incidence of prostate cancer in the world. Because of more limited access to care and possibly lower awareness of risk, Blacks are more likely to be diagnosed at an advanced stage of disease, and they are nearly twice as likely to die of their disease compared to their white counterparts. Although few readers will have Mr. Becker's ability to travel around the country for unlimited consults, you can get good care wherever you are. You need to select your treatment and your treating physician based upon the best available information. The ability of Mr. Becker to use enormous resources made him a more informed patient. This did not help him receive optimal medical treatment in a timely manner. More than six months after I first saw him he had yet to decide on any definitive treatment.

My advice to you, then, is to learn as much as you can in a timely fashion to understand and evaluate the treatment recommendations you are given. This book is designed to provide all the information you need, but a list of recommended readings is included if you are inspired or interested to learn more. Information on finding support groups and on obtaining access to investigational (nonstandard) treatments is also included.

Whatever the stage of your cancer and whatever prognosis you are given, you have a need to know and to understand. Do not *deny* the need for treatment, do not *despair* of getting appropriate treatment, and do not *delay* in seeking that treatment!

2

CANCER AND THE PROSTATE

A FEW WORDS ABOUT CANCER

The word *cancer* arouses fear, shock, and sometimes despair for the individual who hears it from his doctor, and for his family. Nearly everyone has friends and family members who have been given a diagnosis of cancer and survived or succumbed. What is cancer and why is it so common? Why are some cancers much more lethal than others?

Cancer, quite simply, is a collection of abnormal cells that have forgotten how to die. Normally, most types of cells live only a short period of time and are replenished by new cells. Skin cells last just a few weeks, and the cells lining the intestines are also continually dying and being replaced. The cells that die do not produce their own replacements. Instead, this task is performed by "stem" cells that divide to produce two "daughter" cells. The white and red blood cells also have short life spans, and it is the job of the bone marrow to form new white blood cells on a daily basis. Special signals within and between cells communicate that it is time to die or that new replacement cells are needed. This orderly process of continual cell loss and replacement is known as "programmed cell death," or apoptosis.

Cancer cells, unlike healthy normal cells, are "immortal."

While individual cancer cells may disintegrate with age, they are each capable of multiplying indefinitely by cloning themselves. In fact, in many if not all cases, the millions of cells in a tumor all arise from a single abnormal cell. In a cancer, the "replacement" cells vastly outnumber the cells that are lost by normal aging processes. This is the basic abnormality of a cancer. There is an actual increase in the volume and the mass of cells that live in a specific organ.

It may well be the case that many or most of us harbor cancer cells at some point in our lives that are never detected and never grow to a size to do us harm. Some cancers are "latent" or "quiescent"—for some unknown reason, the cells do not multiply or do so quite slowly. Our immune systems may be able to eliminate a small burden of cancer cells or at least curb many cancers' growth so that they never cause symptoms. Prostate cancer, as already mentioned, was long considered to be a latent, very slow-growing cancer that rarely caused death. Autopsies of men who died of other causes have shown that about one-third of men over age fifty have some cancerous cells in their prostate. That incidence increases steadily with age, so that 90 percent of men over ninety have such cells.

WHEN CANCER SPREADS

In addition to their immortality, the other unique feature of cancer cells is their ability to detach themselves from their original site and travel to other parts of the body. This is a complex biological process that is just beginning to be understood. Under normal circumstances, a liver cell is confined to the liver, a stomach cell to the stomach, and a prostate cell to the prostate. When a cell of any of these organs becomes cancerous, it acquires the ability to leave its "birthplace" and take up residence in other parts of the body. This ability to shed cells and establish satellite or daughter cancer colonies in other parts of the body is know as the process of *metastasis*.

Not all cancers are equally able or inclined to spread, and different types of cancer tend to metastasize to particular tissues or organs. Prostate cancer, when it metastasizes, spreads most commonly to the bones, and very rarely to the lungs or liver. We are now beginning to understand how and why different cancers metastasize selectively, information that aids in devising strategies to help prevent the metastases of all cancer.

Once the diagnosis of prostate cancer has been made, all subsequent studies and tests are directed at trying to determine whether the cancer has metastasized. When cancer cells are shed from the primary tumor site, it is common for some of them to find their way to the neighboring lymph nodes, which are part of the immune system that attempts to fight the spread of the abnormal cells. For this reason, a number of the lymph nodes in the pelvis are removed and examined to help determine the extent of the cancer. Since prostate cancer typically spreads to the skeletal bones (particularly the hip and lower back), patients diagnosed with prostate cancer usually undergo bone scans and other tests that look for signs of cancer in the bones. If the lymph nodes are negative and there are no cancerous abnormalities detected in the bones, then it is possible to eliminate the cancer with localized treatment—either surgery or radiation therapy. This means that you, the patient, have a good chance of being cured of your cancer.

If some of the tests performed suggest the presence of metastases outside the prostate gland, then *systemic* rather than *local* treatment is required. Many patients who are told that they have, or may have, metastatic cancer do not understand why the prostate is not removed, since it is the source of the problem. But if the cancer has spread, treatment must be *systemic,* affecting the whole body, both the areas where cancer has been detected and the areas where it may be lurking. Removing the prostate will not eliminate or cure the cancer, and the surgery has too many possible complications to justify performing it when the cancer has already metastasized.

CURABLE VERSUS INCURABLE

Prostate cancer that is still confined to the prostate is considered "curable." Prostate cancer that has metastasized to the lymph nodes or the bones is considered "incurable." This is a judgment and a term that is sometimes callously stated to devastated patients and families by their physicians. Patients often equate the term "incurable" with terminal cancer and impending death. What the term "incurable" really means is that the treatments available are not going to be able to rid the patient of every last cancer cell in his body. As awful as this fact may seem to you and your family if you hear these words from your doctor, it is totally compatible with a long life span and the ability to enjoy years of normal life.

Incurable should not be misinterpreted as meaning untreatable. We routinely treat patients whom we know we can't cure, but these treatments can greatly improve the quality and quantity of life, controlling the cancer for long periods of time. If you are told your cancer is incurable, you should take care of your estate and succession planning, yet understand that you may have a number of years, as many as ten or fifteen, of life ahead of you. You may well be the victim of another illness or accident before this incurable cancer can no longer be treated.

"Curable" can also be misunderstood. We often talk about the five-year cure rate, meaning the number of patients who are cancer-free five years after treatment. While the five-year mark is a very important milestone for you and your family and something to be celebrated, there is nothing magical about the five-year anniversary. If a small number of cancer cells survive treatment, they may begin to multiply at some point five, ten, or even fifteen years in the future. In this case the cancer has "recurred," requiring another round of treatment.

In general, we consider that a person has been "cured" of cancer if, after treatment, he or she lives the same number of years as the average cancer-free individual of the same age.

ABOUT THE PROSTATE

The prostate is usually described as resembling a walnut in size and shape (see Figure 1). It is located deep in the

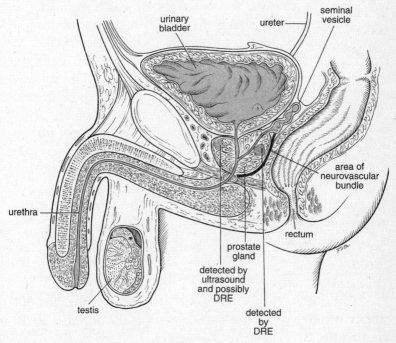

Figure 1

lower pelvis and can be felt (palpated) through the wall of the rectum by the physician during a physical examination. It lies below the urinary bladder and surrounds the urethra, a thin tube resembling a miniature straw. It is through this thin tube that urine passes from the bladder into the penis and out of the body. When the prostate enlarges because of BPH or cancer, it squeezes the urethra and causes problems with urinating.

Some kind of "prostate problem" is almost universal in older men. It is estimated, for example, that by age eighty, 80 percent of all men have noncancerous prostate enlargement—called benign prostate hypertrophy, benign prostate hyperplasia, or BPH for short. Infections of the prostate are also common.

Since the prostate causes so much trouble, you might well wonder what it's good for. It's a gland, which means it can synthesize and secrete into the bloodstream hormones and other chemicals. Important glands include the thyroid, located in the neck, which secretes thyroid hormone, important in helping regulate the body's metabolism. The adrenal gland, located in the back of the abdomen, just above the kidneys, secretes into the bloodstream a number of important steroids and hormones, including the well-known "adrenaline," which helps the body react to stress and to emergencies. There are other types of glands that secrete substances that do not normally enter the bloodstream. The digestive glands, for example, secrete enzymes into the intestines or gut that help the digestive process.

The prostate is considered to be a gland because it secretes many different substances, some of which reach the bloodstream, while some are contributed to the semen at the time of ejaculation, along with secretions of the seminal vesicles, a pair of tubular sacs that lie at the top of the prostate gland. With prostate cancer, BPH, and infection of the prostate, secretion of some of these substances increases.

This is why tests that measure blood levels for two of these substances, acid phosphatase and prostate-specific antigen (PSA), can be used to detect or to monitor disease of the prostate. The secretions contributed by the prostate to the semen apparently help to maintain an appropriate environment for the sperm, improving their survival time after ejaculation. Seen under a microscope, the prostate also has structures and cell types that are characteristic of glands, and so it is called a gland, even though its functions are still rather mysterious.

You may want to know more about the anatomy or structure of the prostate, particularly if you have localized cancer and are considering surgery to remove the prostate (prostatectomy).

The prostate is divided into two lobes—a right and a left—enclosed in a fibrous capsule. This capsule serves as a natural boundary that helps to contain the cancer, but extension of the cancer to the seminal vesicles or the base of the bladder does occur. The lower, wider part of the gland is referred to as the base, and the narrow topmost portion closest to the anus is called the apex. If a prostatectomy is performed, you can expect to be told afterward which lobes or sections showed disease, and whether the margins or borders of the removed prostate are positive (showing cancerous areas) or negative (not involved in the cancer). If the margins are positive, further treatment may be needed to eliminate cancer that may have spread to surrounding structures. If you are told that the margins are negative and there were no signs of spread when the lymph nodes were biopsied, chances are good that your prostatectomy has eliminated the cancer.

For convenience in describing the location of cancers and other problems, the prostate is usually divided into three sectors: the central, transitional, and peripheral zones. The transitional (inner) zone surrounds the urethra and is the tissue causing most of the problems in BPH. Biopsies most often sample the peripheral zone, which is the zone the physician can feel with a gloved finger in a rectal examination and also the zone most often involved in prostate cancer.

PROSTATE ENLARGEMENT AND URINATION

The urinary bladder is a muscular sac that has balloon-like qualities. It stores urine made in the kidney until it can be eliminated from the body. When a certain amount of expansion has occurred in this muscular sac, specialized nerve connections signal that it is time to urinate. Once emptied, the bladder contracts and readies itself to start collecting urine again.

When the prostate gland gets larger, as it invariably does as men age, there may be pressure on the urethra where it passes through the prostate, causing a reduced urinary flow. Nearly every man over the age of forty-five or fifty may notice a mild to moderate decrease in the force of the urinary stream. This is normal, and probably reflects a mild enlargement of the gland pressing on the urethra. A decrease in the force of the stream is called, quite simply, decreased urinary stream.

Imagine for a moment that the normally shaped prostate gland has enlarged even more. As it enlarges, it pushes up on the bottom of the bladder. This pressure in turn may decrease the capacity of the bladder to hold urine. The space which the enlarged prostate gland has taken over now cannot be occupied by urine, and the result is that you have to urinate more frequently. Men who would urinate every five to six hours now find themselves having to go to the bathroom every two or three hours, or even every hour. This effect of prostate enlargement is called urinary frequency, or simply frequency. Although not completely understood, when this situation occurs, the bladder fills up more rapidly and the urge to urinate is quite strong. This sensation is called urgency. Another consequence of an enlarging prostate gland is difficulty in starting the stream of urine. You may be standing at the toilet for several minutes before the stream begins. This phenomenon is called hesitancy.

You may begin getting up in the middle of the night to urinate because of the enlargement of the prostate gland and the bladder's reduced capacity to hold urine. A pattern of nighttime urination is called "nocturia." It may occur once a night in mild forms, while in more severe forms, patients may have three to six episodes of nocturia interrupting their sleep. An enlarged prostate may also result in a feeling that the bladder has not completely emptied itself. In other words, minutes after urinating, you may feel as though you have to go to the bathroom again. Dribbling after urinating is also common.

All of the symptoms just described—decreased stream, frequency, urgency, hesitancy, nocturia, incomplete emptying, and dribbling—can indicate that there may be some enlargement of the prostate gland, infection, or problems in other areas of the urinary tract, such as the bladder. These common symptoms of prostate problems are known collectively as *prostatism*. BPH is the most common cause of these symptoms. It can coexist with prostate cancer, and sometimes patients initially believed to have BPH turn out to have cancer.

CANCER IN AND OF THE PROSTATE

Cancer is not one disease but many. The different diseases of cancer are identified by both the type of cell from which they develop, and the organ in which they originate. Most prostate cancers are a type called adenocarcinoma, which means that they began from glandular cells within the prostate gland. There are other rarer types of prostate cancer, developing from other cell types in the prostate. Because these are so uncommon, we will use the shorter and simpler term *prostate cancer* to mean *prostate adenocarcinoma*. You will also encounter the word *carcinoma*, a more general term for the class of cancers that includes adenocarcinoma.

One of the most confusing areas for many patients and their families is the way cancer that has spread to other areas is described. Prostate cancer that has metastasized to the bones is technically called prostate cancer with bone metastases. It is not bone cancer, as many patients think. The term bone cancer means that the cancer in the bone originated from the bone, and did not get there from another organ. Likewise, prostate cancer that has spread to the lymph nodes is not lymph-node cancer. Lymph-node cancer is a totally different type of cancer, usually called lymphoma, and bears no relationship to prostate cancer.

These are not just hair-splitting distinctions because the origin of a cancer has real significance for treatment and prognosis. Different types of cancer tend to have different life histories and may be more or less sensitive to specific treatment approaches. However, because cancer cells mutate very readily, making them unpredictable and capable of rapid transformations, tumors arising from the same cell type and the same organ can vary considerably in their speed of growth and their resistance to treatment. Prostate cancer is notoriously unpredictable in its progression, for this and other, still unknown reasons.

A CLOSER LOOK AT PROSTATE CANCER

In the prostate gland, the abnormal cancerous cells accumulate to form a small nodule or pea-size collection of cells. The cells become more densely packed, and the consistency of this dense nodule of cells feels abnormal to the gloved finger of the physician during a rectal examination (Figure 1). Because this abnormal collection of cells has a different density, it also reflects sound waves differently during an ultrasound evaluation. For patients with both a physical abnormality and a positive finding on ultrasound, a biopsy is performed to obtain samples of prostate tissue for examination under the microscope by a pathologist. A range of abnormalities—the size, shape, and other physical attributes of cancerous cells—must be identified in the tissue before a diagnosis of cancer can be made.

It is important to realize that it is the microscopic appearance of the cells that provides the definitive diagnosis of cancer. Even though the physician examining someone's prostate gland may have a suspicion that the abnormality is cancer, it is not until tissue is biopsied and examined under the microscope that the actual diagnosis of cancer can be made. There can be a very high index of suspicion that a cancer is present but, again, it is only the microscopic appearance that can definitely establish the diagnosis.

The pathologist looks for abnormal cells and then assesses the degree of abnormality present. Nowadays, genetic markers and molecular fingerprints can also be used to pinpoint the genetic abnormalities. A key term used in this assessment is "differentiation." This word describes the normal process in which new cells mature to acquire their specialized functions within the body. Once a cell has differentiated, it can no longer divide to produce new cells. Cancer cells somehow escape the process of differentiation and are forever able to divide and multiply. When the word differentiation is applied to a cancer, it is used to characterize how closely the cancer still resembles the tissue from which it began. A prostate cancer tissue sample that appears similar to normal glandular structures is usually termed *well differentiated* (see Figure 2).

Figure 2

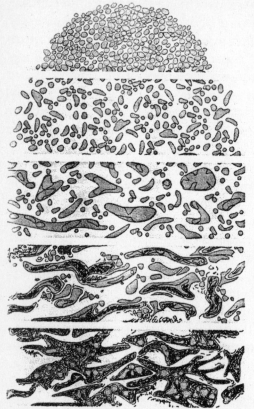

WELL DIFFERENTIATED

1 Glandular (secretory) cells are small, of fairly uniform shape and tightly packed.

2 Cells display more varied and irregular shapes and are loosely packed.

MODERATELY DIFFERENTIATED

3 Cells are even more irregular in size and shape and are more dispersed; some cells are fused, and cell borders are less distinct.

POORLY DIFFERENTIATED

4 Many cells are fused into irregular masses; some cells (*darkly shaded*) have begun to invade the connective tissue that separates cells.

5 Most of the tumor consists of irregular masses that have invaded the connective tissue.

SHAPE, SIZE AND ARRANGEMENT of cancerous cells in the prostate gland are often examined for clues to a tumor's virulence. Well-differentiated tumors (*top two panels*)—those that most resemble normal glandular tissue—are thought to behave less aggressively than do less organized, moderately (*middle panel*) or poorly (*bottom two panels*) differentiated tumors. In the grading scheme depicted above (the Gleason system), the degree of differentiation is indicated by a numerical value ranging from 1 to 5. The score for the predominant pattern is often added to that of the next most prevalent pattern to yield a final Gleason score ranging from 2 to 10.

Although cancer cells "clone" themselves over and over again, their genes are unstable and prone to mutate. Over time, as the cancer continues to grow, accumulating mutations can cause the cells of the cancer to take on a more unusual appearance, not resembling any known structures of the tissue in which it had formed. Such a cancer is considered to be a *moderately differentiated* cancer. If the appearance under the microscope becomes more bizarre and unusual and the cells grow in an uncontrolled fashion, not having any resemblance to any tissue, the cancer is usually described as *poorly differentiated* or *anaplastic.*

For prostate cancer specifically, the degree of differentiation generally holds the answer to how well a patient is likely to do. In other words, the prognosis of the patient can be linked to the microscopic appearance of the cancer—not always, but usually. Thus, a patient with a well-differentiated cancer will generally fare better than a patient with a poorly differentiated tumor. We do not know if there is a progression of a well-differentiated cancer into an anaplastic or poorly differentiated cancer over a period of time, though this is often assumed to be the case. Nor do we know if a particular level of differentiation is predetermined at the time a cancer is born. What we do know is the importance of assessing this pathological feature. We also know that smaller tumors tend to be well-differentiated cancers. This is apparently because the smaller number of cells and of cell generations have limited the number of mutations occurring. In contrast, larger tumors more often than not will be moderately or poorly differentiated.

The differentiation of a prostate cancer is so important that specific grading systems have been established to provide uniformity among pathologists diagnosing the disease. In an important series of early studies performed by the Veterans Administration (see Chapter 5), all of the prostate biopsies were "read" or evaluated by one pathologist, Dr. Donald Gleason. He developed a grading system in order to compare and contrast one prostate tissue sample to another. Dr. Gleason could not know how the patients were going to do at the time he read their biopsies, but the VA studies provided long-term follow-up of the patients. When patient-survival information became available in the years that followed, it was discovered that the Gleason readings of poorly differentiated cancer were associated with a shortened survival and a more advanced stage of disease, compared to a longer survival and less advanced disease for well-differentiated cancers.

Dr. Gleason scored the cell differentiation pattern in each prostate biopsy on a scale of 1 to 5. A pattern score of 1 represented the most well-differentiated type of cancer, while a pattern score of 5 represented the most anaplastic type of cancer. In actuality, most biopsies will include a variety of cells in different states of differentiation. For this reason, Gleason would determine the most numerous cancer-cell type present, followed by the next most common type. These two Gleason numbers are referred to as the primary and secondary pattern scores. Using this system, a biopsy might be scored as a "Gleason 3 + 3" or a "Gleason 3 + 4." The most favorable or well-differentiated cancer would be a "Gleason 1 + 1" or combined pattern score of 2, while the most undifferentiated cancer would be a "Gleason 5 + 5" or combined pattern score of 10 (Figure 2).

Using this system to read the prostate biopsy, Dr. Gleason was able to predict how long a patient would survive with a high degree of accuracy. With new treatment modalities this is not the case today, but an accurate pathological assessment is vital to determining the best treatment and the outcome to be expected.

While most pathologists utilize the Gleason scoring system, not all do, and probably do not have to. Oftentimes, the terms "well," "moderately," and "poorly" differentiated are used. These terms usually correspond to combined Gleason scores of 2–4, 5–7, and 8–10, respectively. Likewise, cancers graded as Grade I, II, or III generally have the same meaning. (The importance of the differentiation will come up again when we discuss the management of the patient with a cancer diagnosed as a result of PSA-based screening.)

Table 1. Comparison of Staging Systems for Prostate Cancer

TNM System	Conventional System
T0 No evidence of prostate cancer	
T1 No palpable lesion	Stage A Clinically unsuspected disease
T1a Three or fewer microscopic foci of carcinoma	A1 Focal carcinoma, usually well differentiated
T1b More than three microscopic foci of carcinoma	A2 Diffuse carcinoma, usually poorly differentiated
T1c Cancer detected by PSA elevation	
T2 Tumor clinically present, limited to the prostate gland	Stage B Tumor confined to prostate gland
T2a Tumor 1.5 cm or less in greatest diameter with normal tissue on at least three sides	B1 Small, discrete nodule of one lobe of gland
T2b Tumor more than 1.5 cm in greatest diameter or in more than one lobe of the prostate	B2 Large or multiple nodules or areas of involvement
T3 Tumor invades prostatic apex, seminal vesicle, bladder neck, or is into or beyond prostate capsule, but not fixed	Stage C Tumor localized to the periprostatic area C1 Tumor outside prostatic capsule, estimated weight less than 70 g, seminal vesicles uninvolved
T4 Tumor is fixed or invades adjacent structures other than the structures listed in T3 (above)	C2 Tumor outside prostatic capsule, estimated weight more than 70 g, seminal vesicles involved
N Lymph node metastases	Stage D Metastatic prostate cancer
N1 Metastasis in a single pelvic node, less than 2 cm in greatest dimension	D1 Pelvic lymph node metastases and/or ureteral obstruction causing hydronephrosis
N2 Metastasis in a single pelvic node, more than 2 cm but less than 5 cm in diameter; or multiple lymph node metastases, none greater than 5 cm in greatest dimension	
N3 Metastasis in a single pelvic lymph node greater than 5 cm in diameter	
M Distant metastatic disease	
M1 Bone, soft tissue, organ, or distant lymph node metastases	D2 Bone, soft tissue, organ, or distant lymph node metastases

CANCER STAGING

Once a patient has had the diagnosis of prostate cancer established with a pathological level of differentiation, we next engage in a series of evaluations that have an equally important impact—the determination of the extent of the cancer. Perhaps the most important information of all to obtain, this determines whether the patient will be cured of prostate cancer, or whether he will eventually die from it.

The extent of the cancer—the degree of its advancement—is called its stage.

There are several staging systems for describing the state of advancement of prostate cancer. One commonly used system is shown in Table 1. It subdivides the level of advancement into stages A, B, C, and D, with stage A representing the least advanced disease and D the most advanced. The first three stages are distinguished from one another by the size of the tumors. Stages A, B, and certain stage C disease include cancers that have not spread; they have not spawned new tumor colonies in other tissues away from the prostate gland. Some stage C and all stage D disease consists of tumors that have already spread beyond the prostate capsule either by direct extension (growth into surrounding tissue) or metastases.

Stage A

Stage A cancers are microscopic. These cancers can be divided into two subclasses. Stage A1 cancers are "focal"—confined to one small area of the prostate—and are composed of relatively well-differentiated cancer. There are some obviously cancerous abnormalities in the cells (such as an enlarged cell nucleus) seen under the pathologist's microscope, but the tumor cells are of uniform size and closely packed, like healthy gland cells. Stage A2 cancers are more diffuse or disseminated (found in more of the tissue examined), consist of moderately to poorly differentiated tissue, or display both characteristics. Multiple tumor sites in the prostate gland or poor differentiation implies that the cancer is likely to behave aggressively—growing rapidly or shedding cancerous cells into the bloodstream.

A stage A1 cancer is one picked up incidentally at the time of transurethral resection of the prostate (TURP) for apparently benign enlargement of the prostate gland (BPH). When the "chips" of removed tissue are examined by the pathologist, microscopic amounts of cancer, usually well differentiated (Gleason combined pattern score of 4 or less), are seen. The transurethral resection was generally all the treatment that was called for, and more often than not the patient did not suffer further from the cancer. With longer term follow-up of ten to fifteen years, we now know that about 15 percent of these stage A1 patients show some form of progressive disease, with about 8 percent of the patients dying of prostate cancer. Because this type of long-term follow-up data is available, today patients can be in a better position to determine whether they want further treatment if a stage A1 cancer is detected. Currently, we do not have the same type of long-term follow-up or outcome studies for cancers detected by PSA-based screening (so-called T1c cancers, discussed below).

Patients with stage A2 disease generally have more cancer in the gland, with a higher Gleason score. In a proportion of patients, these cancers may have spread to the lymph node areas. Thus most if not all A2 patients will end up with some form of treatment.

Stage B

Stage B cancers are palpable—meaning large enough to be felt as a nodule or hardening in the peripheral zone of the prostate gland during a rectal examination, which is generally how they are diagnosed. They usually do not cause any symptoms or discomfort, although some men may have urinary symptoms that were believed to be related to BPH. B1 designates a small nodule found only on one lobe, while large or multiple nodules are usually staged as B2 disease. All stage B tumors are those still localized to the gland, with no metastases or direct extension to surrounding tissue. However, at the time of surgery, they are often found to be more extensive—pointing to a limitation in our ability to stage cancer "clinically" before treatment is undertaken.

Stage C

Stage C tumors have spread through most or all of the prostate gland, making it rock hard, and have pushed past the borders of the prostate into surrounding structures. C1 is the category often used for disease that has spread outside the prostate capsule but not to the seminal vesicles, while C2 and C3 describe cancer that is believed to have spread to involve the seminal vesicles. Patients who have stage C cancers are often diagnosed after urinary symptoms cause them to seek medical help.

If the cancer has spread into the seminal vesicles adjacent to the prostate, the patient is still classified as having stage C disease, but often he will soon develop evidence of spread to distant organs. For this reason, some patients with stage C2 or C3 cancer will be treated as though they in fact have metastatic or stage D disease.

Stage D

Stage D is cancer that has metastasized to the lymph nodes or bone, or possibly other tissues as well. D1 is the substage used to describe patients who have cancerous cells detected in their lymph nodes, while D2 describes those who have actual metastases in the bone or sometimes other tissues. Two other subcategories are sometimes mentioned. D0 is used for patients whose only evidence of stage D metastatic disease is an elevated acid phosphatase level, which is a marker for metastatic prostate cancer. Stage D3 is sometimes used to describe metastatic prostate cancer that has become resistant (refractory) to hormonal therapy.

You must understand that "D" does not stand for death. Men with stage D1 disease many times live out normal lives if they receive appropriate and timely treatment. Stage D2 disease can also be controlled for long periods of time, sometimes a number of years, before the cancer becomes resistant to our best available treatments and becomes stage D3 disease.

Classifying "PSA" Tumors

Another staging approach often used both in this country and abroad is the TNM system, shown in Table 1 on page 35. The acronym stands for Tumor, Nodes, and Metastases. The T classification is based on the size of the cancer. The N status is assigned according to whether there is lymph-node involvement. The M classification is then assigned, depending upon whether there has been distant spread to portions of the body outside the prostate gland.

While both systems are in use, there is one specific situation in which the TNM system is used almost exclusively. The stage of disease referred to as T1c is one of the most commonly diagnosed stages of prostate cancer in the 1990s. This stage describes cancer diagnosed in a patient who is totally without symptoms but who has an elevated PSA level on a routine screening. Unlike patients who have stage A1 cancer, T1c patients have no specific urinary complaints even referable to BPH. For these patients, there will be no abnormalities evident with a physical examination or ultrasound. However, a biopsy of the prostate gland, prompted by the abnormal PSA, will reveal the presence of cancer.

In other words, until we began doing routine PSA screening just a few years ago, men who had T1c disease were never diagnosed. Either their cancer grew until it began causing urinary symptoms and was then diagnosed, or their cancer never advanced to the point where it caused symptoms, and they died "with" rather than "of" prostate cancer. Because the diagnosis of T1c cancer is so new, we don't yet know what the long-term prognosis for these patients will be if a policy of "watchful waiting" is taken in the belief that their disease is a latent "die with" cancer.

We do know, however, what the typical Gleason patterns and other biopsy findings are for these T1c cancers. We can attempt to compare and contrast these findings with the long-term outcomes of patients who had similar pathological findings, but whose cancers were not detected by PSA-based screening. Several major studies have now evaluated the detailed pathological findings of patients who were treated for prostate cancer detected after PSA screening. In one study, the pathology results were compared to a group of men who sought medical attention because of urinary symptoms. This study compared differences in cancer stages of patients detected at the time of symptoms to those detected without symptoms.

These studies demonstrated that PSA-based screening detected more organ-confined cancers compared to those cancers in a symptomatic group of patients. More cancers that fell into the definition of latent cancers were also detected in the "screened" group compared to the symptomatic group. However, the majority of the cancers detected by PSA-based screening had characteristics which would predict them to be clinically important cancers. Between 88 percent and 94 percent of the cancers were moderately or poorly differentiated cancers (Gleason combined score greater than 5) and the cancers were multifocal, meaning that they were present in multiple parts of the gland.

UNCERTAINTIES OF STAGING

To stage tumors clinically, physicians first combine the information gleaned from the rectal examination and the ultrasound with information provided by other noninvasive tests described in Chapter 3. For example, a CT (computed tomography) scan of the abdomen and pelvis may be carried out to search for evidence of cancer in the lymph nodes. If metastases are a possibility, a bone scan will look for the presence of cancerous deposits in the bones. Magnetic resonance imaging (MRI) can help determine if the prostate gland tumor has spread locally beyond the prostate capsule. To determine the Gleason grade, as well as estimate the tumor extent within the gland, samples of prostate tissue obtained by needle biopsy are examined under the microscope. These evaluations all help to assign a "clinical" stage to the patient.

Unfortunately, the diagnostic tests that are utilized to assign a clinical stage are inaccurate in 25 percent to 60 percent of patients initially assigned to stages A2, B, or C. If surgery is the treatment option taken, after some of the pelvic lymph nodes and the prostate are removed and biopsied, these patients may be found to have more advanced cancer. Stage C patients may turn out to have metastatic disease, and men who are believed to have stage B cancers will often have stage C cancers. In short, cancer is often "understaged" clinically (thought to be less advanced) until the surgical staging is done. There is less chance that a patient who has been diagnosed as A1 disease will later be found to have metastatic or "extraprostatic" cancer.

To determine the stage more accurately, physicians may do additional biopsies of the lymph nodes to study the tissue for the presence of metastatic deposits. Unfortunately, this surgical staging technique cannot detect stray cancerous cells that have escaped into the bloodstream and lodged in the bones. Thus, based upon the characteristics of the primary cancer in the prostate gland, some patients who are treated as though they have early-stage cancer will actually have metastatic cancer. For this reason, the PSA level must be monitored after treatment to help identify those individuals who were understaged.

Recent research is helping to discover ways of detecting the smallest number of cancer cells which have escaped from the prostate gland, to improve the accuracy of staging and the correct choice of treatments. New tests using sophisticated molecular techniques can detect a single PSA-producing prostate cell (presumed to be a shed cancer cell, since normal prostate cells do not circulate) among ten million blood cells. However, at this point in time, these tests are regarded as promising but not yet definitive techniques for basing treatment decisions.

Table 2 sets forth the "traditional" treatment choices based upon the stage of the cancer. While I feel obliged to include such a table, I must caution that it is only a guideline, and should not, under any circumstances, be interpreted as giving the treatment plan you should expect or seek. As you continue to read this book, the complexities of selecting the appropriate treatment for you as an individual will become more clear. In other words, there is no simple "cookbook" approach to recommending specific treatments. Hence, my reason for writing this book, and yours for reading it!

Table 2
Typical Therapies for Prostate Cancer

Treatment for prostate cancer is based on the stage to which the disease has advanced. The standard recommendations in the U.S. are listed in the rightmost column. Use of aggressive therapy—radiation or radical prostatectomy (surgery to remove the prostate gland)—for stage A and B disease has become increasingly controversial because some data suggest nontreatment may result in a comparable survival rate or in a better quality of life for certain patients. Those findings, however, are inconclusive and remain a subject of debate.

STAGE OF DISEASE		STANDARD THERAPY
STAGE A MICROSCOPIC CANCER WITHIN PROSTATE GLAND	**A1** Cancer confined to one site and is well differentiated	Observation, radiation or radical prostatectomy
	A2 Cancer occurs in many sites or is moderately to poorly differentiated	Radiation or radical prostatectomy
STAGE B PALPABLE LUMP WITHIN PROSTATE GLAND	**B1** Cancer forms a small, discrete nodule in one lobe of gland	Radiation or radical prostatectomy
	B2 Cancer forms a large nodule or multiple nodules, or it involves both lobes or is moderately to poorly differentiated	
STAGE C LARGE MASS INVOLVING ALL OR MOST OF PROSTATE GLAND	**C1** Cancer occurs as a continuous mass that may have extended somewhat beyond the gland	Radiation; some physicians administer hormonal therapy with radiation
	C2 Larger cancer occurs as a continuous mass that has invaded structures surrounding the gland	
STAGE D METASTATIC TUMOR	**D1** Cancer occurs in the lymph nodes of the pelvis	Hormonal therapy once symptoms arise (or possibly as soon as metastatic deposits are found) and palliative therapy for pain and other discomforts
	D2 Cancer involves tissues beyond the lymph nodes, usually including the bones	
	D3 Treatment resistant prostate cancer	Non-standard therapies

3

DIAGNOSING PROSTATE CANCER

With the development and widespread use of the PSA test, we now have greatly expanded our ability to detect prostate cancer at an early stage, when treatment has a high likelihood of being curative. The PSA test itself, of course, does not diagnose cancer. Rather, it provides one of many clues needed to determine whether cancer may or may not be present.

There are several steps to diagnosing, grading, and staging prostate cancer. The aim is always to obtain the most precise possible information about the individual disease stage while minimizing discomfort and risk for the patient. Some cancers can be accurately assessed with a PSA test, a rectal exam, ultrasound, and a series of needle biopsies of the prostate, but whenever metastases are a possibility, the diagnostic workup is usually more extensive.

Even if you have "been through it already"—your diagnosis has already been made and confirmed by biopsy—I still suggest that you read this and the following chapter thoroughly. Our diagnostic evaluations do not give us 100 percent certainty, and you will later read about a few patients who were told their cancer was much more or much less advanced than it later proved to be. Also, a number of these diagnostic tools are also used for monitoring the success of treatment. You will continue to have PSA and DRE tests, for example, to catch early warning signs of cancer recurrence, so you should know what kind of information these tests provide, and how they should be interpreted.

Figure 3

UNDERSTANDING CLINICAL STAGING OF PROSTATE CANCER
ASSESSING BOTH PROSTATE GLAND AND THE BODY

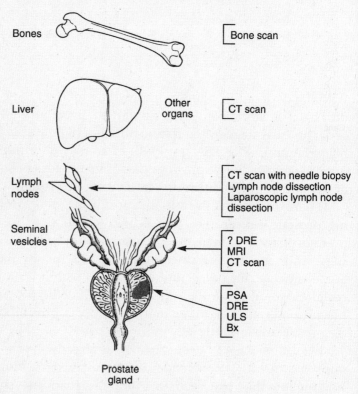

Bones — Bone scan

Liver / Other organs — CT scan

Lymph nodes — CT scan with needle biopsy / Lymph node dissection / Laparoscopic lymph node dissection

Seminal vesicles — ? DRE / MRI / CT scan

— PSA / DRE / ULS / Bx

Prostate gland

Figure 3 indicates the tests used in diagnosing and staging prostate cancer that you may undergo. Each portion of the body may require a different test to assess whether the cancer has spread to that area, thus allowing us to determine the ex-

Figure 4

PATHOLOGICAL STAGING OF PROSTATE CANCER
ASSESSING ONLY THE PROSTATE GLAND AREA

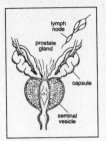

Radical prostatectomy allows the determination of extent of cancer in the prostate gland, prostate capsule, seminal vesicle, and lymph node because these tissues are removed and examined under the microscope.

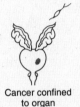

| Cancer confined to organ | Margin positive disease capsular involvement | Regional disease seminal vesicle positive | Positive lymph nodes involved |

tent of the disease. Figure 4 shows the pathological staging that is determined after the radical prostatectomy has been performed and the pathologist has examined the prostate gland and surrounding tissues under the microscope.

PSA—PROSTATE-SPECIFIC ANTIGEN

The prostate has been long known to secrete a variety of chemicals, which can be measured in the bloodstream, that indicate an abnormality. Acid phosphatase, for example, is one such substance that has been known for decades to be associated with prostate cancer as well as a variety of other disorders. Even though acid phosphatase was known to be produced by the prostate gland, it could be detected under circumstances not associated with any prostate gland abnormalities. In other words, its presence was not prostate-gland or prostate-cancer specific.

That has all changed with the advent of the PSA test. Discovered in the late 1970s by researchers at Roswell Park Memorial Hospital, its use in one form or another has been clinically available for nearly fifteen years. In the early 1980s, I would routinely use a PSA test to determine whether a patient who had a diagnosis of cancer based on a lymph node or liver biopsy, in fact had a cancer that originated in the prostate gland. A biopsy of the tissue would be stained with special chemicals to determine whether the cancer cells contained PSA. If they did, this could be taken for strong evidence that the cancer was of prostate gland origin, which had then spread to the liver or lymph node. Such information is critical in trying to determine what kind of treatment program to embark upon.

Today it is easy to measure the actual amount of PSA in the bloodstream, and this serves as the basis for the PSA blood test. Although not known with certainty, most researchers believe that PSA, along with other prostate gland secretions, is needed to maintain the viability of the sperm after ejaculation into the vagina. Whatever its function, we do know that both normal prostate cells and prostate cancer cells are capable of manufacturing PSA, which is also secreted into the bloodstream.

Every male has a certain level of PSA that circulates in the bloodstream. For patients with perfectly normal prostate glands, the level represents a "normal value"—usually said to be under 4.0 ng/ml (nanograms per milliliter). Our estimate of the "normal" range of PSA concentration is constantly being refined and redefined as the laboratory analytic tests become more sophisticated and as we acquire more information from studies of men of all ages with normal and abnormal prostates. New methodologies are being introduced that may have slight variations of the "normal values."

It is important to understand that PSA is prostate-gland

specific, but not prostate-cancer specific. What this means is that the PSA measured in the bloodstream all comes from prostate gland cells. The PSA test works as a screening and monitoring tool because prostate cancer cells generally manufacture more PSA per cell than a normal prostate cell. If the

Figure 5

PSA DENSITY

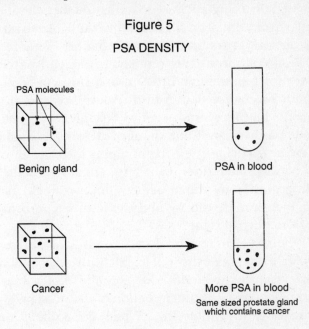

PSA molecules

Benign gland

PSA in blood

Cancer

More PSA in blood

Same sized prostate gland
which contains cancer

blood level is abnormally high, it may signify the presence of cancer in the prostate gland even though the physical exam and the ultrasound-wave test are both normal (Figure 5).

Since both normal and cancerous cells can make PSA, an abnormal value can be due to a normal aging and enlarging prostate gland, trauma to the buttocks or prostate area, prostate infection (prostatitis), or prostate cancer. PSA is also elevated following any activity or exercise that results in stress to the rectum or the perineum (the area between the anus and the scrotum). For example, PSA is often slightly elevated after a DRE, a biopsy, sexual intercourse, or exercise.

Strenuous exercise that puts stress on the buttocks, such as bicycling, can raise the PSA level substantially. A level of 70 ng/ml was reported in a man who experienced pelvic trauma while crewing on a sailing vessel. Because of these variables, a diagnosis or a treatment decision should never be based on a single PSA test result, however elevated.

To avoid the need for repeating the PSA test, you might want to avoid strenuous activities that are likely to increase the PSA level for seven to ten days before you go to see your doctor for follow-up and PSA monitoring. An acquaintance of mine was biopsied after his PSA level was measured as 5.6 ng/ml. The biopsy was negative but the PSA remained elevated and there was some thought of doing a second biopsy. When he told me these facts, along with the information that he was a bike rider, I suggested that he abstain from bicycling and from sexual activity for two weeks before his next PSA test. He did so, and the level was returned as 3.5 ng/ml, a normal value.

Whenever an abnormal PSA result is obtained, it is important to confirm the test result with a second value. In many instances, patients with elevated PSA values will be treated for prostatitis (an infection of the prostate gland that is treated with antibiotics). When the value is repeated, chances are good that the PSA will come back down to normal if it was due to infection. While this does not guarantee the absence of cancer, it does suggest that the elevation was due to the infection.

If you travel or change physicians during the course of your evaluation and treatment, you should know that PSA tests are not all the same. Progress is being made to establish a standard, but until that is achieved, different test manufacturers measure PSA slightly differently. Depending upon the "brand" of PSA test used, normal ranges are between 0–2.8 or 0–3.4 or 0–4.0. Chapter 4 provides more information on the subtleties of interpreting the information provided by the PSA test.

DRE—DIGITAL RECTAL EXAMINATION

For the DRE, the physician inserts a gloved finger into the rectum, where the prostate can be felt (palpated) through the rectal wall. (Here the word *digital* simply means "using a finger," not "electronic"!) Even though the prostate gland is located under the urinary bladder, its rearmost portions can be felt through the rectum during a DRE. The examining finger can feel some, but not all, of the gland—glandular consistency, abnormal contour, or areas of hardness can usually be appreciated. A very enlarged or rock-hard gland suggests certain possibilities in the diagnosis. A rubbery gland or gland of softer consistency indicates another set of diagnoses. After the rectal exam, which is also a generally good method to detect abnormalities of the rectum, the physician may feel that the exam should be complemented with other tests, such as ultrasound, to get a better "look" at the gland and gain more information about its functioning.

It had been taught for decades that the most sensitive manner in which to detect prostate cancer was by means of the digital rectal examination. With the development of the PSA test and transrectal ultrasound (TRUS), this is no longer the case. A series of studies have been done comparing the sensitivity and reliability of PSA screening and DRE in detecting prostate cancer in symptom-free (asymptomatic) men over the age of fifty. Based upon several thousand patients, the findings suggested that the PSA test is a better screening procedure in detecting prostate cancer. PSA picked up nearly 30 percent of cancers that were not detectable by DRE alone. DRE was also able to detect cancers that were missed by PSA screening, but the proportion was less. However, today both tests should be performed.

Some physicians are overconfident of their ability to detect any and all significant prostate cancers through the rectal exam. If your physician dismisses an abnormal PSA because the physical exam is normal, you would be well advised to seek another opinion.

TRUS—TRANSRECTAL ULTRASOUND

The next diagnostic test to be performed is usually an ultrasound examination of the prostate gland. This is a sound-wave test in which an instrument (called a probe) is inserted into the rectal area, and sound waves are given off that pass through the rectum (transrectal) to neighboring organs. The probe allows the physician (a radiologist or a specially trained urologist) to aim the sound waves at the prostate. A monitor displays and records the reflections or echoes of those sound waves in the form of an image of the organ.

The TRUS or transrectal ultrasound is helpful in examining specific abnormalities that are first detected on DRE, but it also provides very important information about abnormalities that cannot be detected on physical examination of the gland. Because of the density or thickness of the cancerous tissue, fewer or smaller sound waves (echoes) are reflected by it and the composite image formed by ultrasound is different. A "hypoechoic" abnormality appearing on TRUS raises the possibility of cancer. This is not always the case, however, as a variety of benign (noncancerous) conditions can give a similar appearance.

A noteworthy advance of the ultrasound test has been in helping identify prostate problems when there is a high suspicion that cancer may be present but there are no physical abnormalities. The suspicion of such a cancer may be based on an abnormal PSA test. Using TRUS here can often identify abnormalities, which may then be biopsied.

There is also another excellent and important reason for performing TRUS—it can "see" into areas of the prostate gland that are not accessible by the examining finger and allows nearly all areas of the prostate to be assessed. In other words, it adds a greater dimension to the examination. It can also visualize surrounding anatomic structures located near the prostate gland, such as the tubes that store semen and sperm. If the ultrasound test that has identified an abnormality suggestive of a possible cancer and the physical examination using the DRE correlate with one another, it is very likely that the abnormal area will be biopsied.

TRUS is also used to help guide the physician doing a needle biopsy of the prostate. If, for example, the physical abnormality of the gland is not easily identified, it may be difficult to pinpoint exactly where to biopsy. When the ultrasound is more precise in outlining the abnormality, the biopsy procedure can be more accurate, allowing the physician to aim the needle at the ultrasound target. This type of procedure is called an ultrasound-guided biopsy.

BIOPSY OF THE PROSTATE GLAND

For patients with a physical abnormality and/or a positive finding on ultrasound, a biopsy of the prostate is performed to obtain small tissue or cell samples that can be examined under the microscope by a pathologist. If the TRUS suggests the possibility of spread beyond the prostate capsule, the physician may decide to do an ultrasound-guided biopsy that samples tissue not only from the gland itself but from the seminal vesicles and other neighboring (periprostatic) tissues. The risk of complications seems to be no greater with the extraprostatic ("beyond the prostate") sampling, and the additional information obtained can be critical to accurate staging of the cancer.

Often, when the PSA is quite elevated but there is no abnormality found by TRUS or DRE, a "blind" biopsy is performed, in which the physician takes tissue samples more or less randomly, usually three or four from each of the two lobes of the prostate gland. The term "blind biopsy" simply means that the physician is not targeting a known abnormality but rather just getting samples of prostate tissue for analysis.

To do a biopsy, the physician places a hollow, spring-loaded needle in the rectum, aiming it at prostate gland abnormalities identified by DRE or TRUS and using it to draw a small core of tissue from the prostate. Occasionally, an ultrasound-guided biopsy is done by passing the needle through the perineum, the area between the anus and the scrotum. In either case, the procedure is quick and for most patients fairly painless, or associated with only mild pain.

Rather than sampling an entire piece of tissue, the doctor sometimes inserts a smaller needle into the prostate gland and applies suction to pull a sample into the needle. What is obtained here are individual cells rather than a three-dimensional piece of prostate tissue. A specialized pathologist, called a cytopathologist, examines these individual cells under the microscope and can usually tell if any are cancer cells. This procedure, called an "aspiration biopsy" or "fine-needle aspirate," provides less valuable information, but is also less uncomfortable for the patient with perhaps less risk of infection or bleeding. In certain circumstances the information obtained from a fine-needle aspirate is sufficient and adequate to plan treatment.

A properly performed biopsy provides the most definitive information on whether a cancer is or is not present. However, it is an invasive procedure and there is a risk of complications. Because the needle doing the biopsy has to pass through the rectum, there is always a possibility that bacteria from the rectum can be introduced at the time of the biopsy. These bacteria can gain access to the bloodstream, at which point the patient could become extremely ill, or they can lodge in the prostate gland itself. Fortunately, these complications can be minimized by the appropriate use of antibiotics; cleansing enemas are sometimes administered as well. Shaking chills and the development of a fever after a biopsy demands immediate medical attention, sometimes requiring hospitalization and intravenous antibiotics. It is not uncommon to find blood in the semen or ejaculate after a biopsy. This is very distressing for the patient who has not been warned that it may occur. It is quite minor and is usually resolved within a week or two. On rare occasions, there may be some disturbances in ejaculatory function following the biopsy, but this is unusual.

ENDORECTAL COIL MRI

There is a new MRI-based diagnostic procedure that can improve our ability to assess cancers that may have spread by direct extension to surrounding tissue such as the seminal vesicles, the prostatic capsule, the prostate urethra, or the base of the bladder. This can be very important information for deciding whether prostate surgery alone is likely to remove the entire cancer and cure the patient.

Magnetic resonance imaging (MRI) has been most often used to assess head injuries and brain disorders. Because the standard MRI images the whole body, organs deep within the abdomen or pelvis (such as the prostate) could not as readily be viewed using magnetic imaging technology. Now the coil used to generate a magnetic field can be placed in the rectum (endorectal) for an "up close and personal" view of the prostate and surrounding tissue, including the seminal vesicles. Cancerous cells have a distinct magnetic "spin" and this shows up in the image.

BONE SCAN

You will remember that prostate cancer, when it metastasizes, is commonly found in skeletal bone, and rarely in the liver or other organs. For this reason, when the PSA is quite elevated or the DRE and ultrasound suggest a large, aggressive tumor, the bones must be evaluated for signs of cancer. My policy is to obtain a bone scan even when metastates are not suspected as a baseline evaluation in case there is disease recurrence or progression at some point in the future.

A bone scan is a nuclear medicine procedure in which a small tracer amount of a radioactive substance is injected into the patient. This substance is taken up by areas where the bone is growing or repairing itself. In an active cancer, you will remember, cells are dividing and multiplying at a much higher rate than in normal tissue. An area of rapid cell growth can be detected as a "hot spot" on the scan, using a special camera that detects the amount of gamma radiation coming from the bone. If you are told your bone scan is "abnormal," you need to know that not all abnormalities on the bone scan are due to metastatic cancer, and indeed most can be explained by some other cause. A bone scan interpreted as revealing cancer is said to be "positive."

Conventional X-rays generally are not very helpful in imaging or diagnosing prostate cancer metastases that are still asymptomatic (causing no pain). However, when there is a suspicious area on the bone scan, it is useful to obtain regular X-rays of the area to see what they show. The reasoning here is based on the fact that the bone scan is more likely to become positive and show abnormal areas secondary to cancer before the regular X-rays will. If the bone scan is definitely abnormal and the plain X-ray shows no evidence of abnormalities, it is another evidence suggesting that the bone scan may have detected a colony of cancer cells. If, however, there is an abnormality on the X-ray that matches the abnormal area on the bone scan, the radiologist may conclude that the positive bone scan is due to arthritis or some other benign condition of the bone that is readily detected by both X-ray and bone scans.

CT SCAN—
COMPUTERIZED TOMOGRAPHY

If the prostate biopsy is "positive"—found to contain cancer—then other diagnostic studies may be required to determine if the cancer has metastasized. When and if a prostate cancer sheds cells with the potential to establish new colonies of cancer cells in the bones or other organs, these cells are often picked up by small vessels called lymphatics, which carry them to lymph nodes.

The lymph nodes serve as a defense mechanism for the body to try and ward off or contain foreign "invaders." In the case of infections, lymph nodes can drain the infected area and pick up bacteria, which explains the swollen neck lymph nodes that can accompany a sore throat. In the case of cancer cells, the lymph nodes can attempt to wall off a cancer cell from wandering throughout the body. Sometimes the shed cancer cells overwhelm this defense mechanism and establish a small colony within the lymph nodes. Either way, the presence of cancer cells in one or more lymph nodes is an indication that the cancer requires systemic, not just local treatment.

Depending upon the location of the tissue from which the cancer arises, certain lymph nodes may become enlarged. Our bodies have regional stations in which the lymph nodes reside, each designed to serve a different "territory." In the case of the prostate gland, the territory that is most likely to be challenged by the shed cancer cell is located in the pelvis and the back of the abdomen. Luckily, there are abundant lymph nodes in these areas that can serve as a primary line of defense to slow or prevent cancer spread.

In many instances, a determination of the lymph node status becomes a very important portion of the evaluation. The most simple way in which to see if the lymph nodes are enlarged is to perform a specialized X-ray test known as a pelvic-abdominal CT scan, or sometimes "CAT scan" (computerized axial tomography). A specialized X-ray machine takes images at different planes or "slices" of a tissue, then uses computer enhancement capabilities to form a composite image of the organ being studied.

The information obtained from a CT scan is valuable in determining whether the cancer has spread beyond the limits of the prostate gland. We can determine whether the lymph nodes are enlarged (which is suggestive but not 100 percent definitive for the presence of cancer), and also look for signs that prostate cancer has spread to other parts of the body. Another reason for performing a CT scan is to get some information on the function of the kidneys.

In the past, many times when men with prostate cancer were diagnosed with advanced forms of the disease, it was common for enlarged lymph nodes to cause additional blockage of the urine flow from the kidneys to the bladder. If this occurred, the kidneys and the tubes from the kidneys could become swollen and dilated. This ballooning of the tubes can be detected by either special X-rays of the kidneys, or with the CT scan. Although this type of condition is less common today, if present, it does require more urgent treatment to restore kidney function and preserve the kidneys.

If the CT scan shows swollen or enlarged lymph nodes, that finding strongly suggests cancer may be present in those nodes, making it "node-positive" disease. However, there are other reasons for swollen nodes. In order to be sure, a biopsy of those lymph nodes which appear abnormal on the CT scan is often advisable.

BIOPSY OF THE LYMPH NODES

If the pathologist's report, the CT scan, and other diagnostic information suggest that the cancer may have metastasized, then it is often necessary to biopsy the lymph nodes. This can be done as a surgical operation in which a number of lymph nodes are removed and examined, through a laporoscope, or as a needle biopsy, which is a less invasive procedure that provides less definitive information.

Biopsy at the Time of Prostate Surgery

The first, most common procedure is to proceed on the assumption that the prostate cancer is localized and plan to remove the prostate gland surgically in a radical prostatectomy. However, before the surgery is actually performed, the surgeon makes an incision, exposes the area of the lymph nodes, snips off a piece of the lymph node tissue, and gives it to the pathologist. A "frozen section" of the nodal tissue is prepared, which allows the pathologist to look at the tissue under the microscope immediately. All this is done while you are still on the operating-room table under general anesthesia. The entire procedure of waiting for the interpretation of the frozen section takes about fifteen to thirty minutes.

If the pathologist finds no cancer in the lymph node tissue, the surgeon, with permission received from you ahead of time, proceeds with the radical prostatectomy. If, however, there is evidence of cancer spread to the lymph nodes, the surgeon, again with your agreement in advance, will usually stop the operation, without having removed the prostate gland.

This is the standard procedure in these situations, because if the lymph nodes are positive for cancer, removing the prostate will not cure the cancer. Even though the shed cancer cells seem to be walled off and limited to the area of the lymph nodes, over a period of time additional cancer cells are very likely to appear in other parts of the body. Removing the prostate gland and/or the lymph nodes does not seem to have an effect on the rate at which these other metastatic cancers occur in the body. The mere fact that the cancer cells have gained access to the lymph nodes indicates that the cancer has become more widespread, even though at the time of surgery we cannot detect the spread. The cancer is now considered systemic, that is, no longer localized or confined to a specific area that would allow complete removal and possible cure.

A very similar procedure is followed in treating women with breast cancer, for much the same reasons. Following diagnosis of a cancerous breast lump, a sampling of the "regional" lymph nodes is undertaken. In the case of breast disease, these regional lymph nodes are located under the armpit, not in the groin, as they are for prostate cancer. If these armpit lymph nodes contain cancer, the patient is felt to have systemic disease that is undetectable by our current diagnostic modalities.

Patients with positive lymph nodes are very likely to have "micrometastatic" disease—cancer cells that are lodged throughout the body, but have not grown to sufficient size to be detectable or visible by physical examination or X-ray tests. The practical meaning for patients, both those diagnosed with prostate cancer and breast cancer with positive nodes, is that the cancer is unlikely to be cured by removal of only the organ in which the cancer originated.

Thus the patient who is found to have positive nodes at the time of contemplated radical prostatectomy will usually not have the prostate removed. This patient is statistically more likely to suffer problems from the spread of his prostate cancer to other areas of the body. So, it has been argued, why subject the patient to a long and intensive operation if the operation is unlikely to result in curing the patient of his cancer. In some special cases the radical prostatectomy will still be performed when the lymph nodes are found to be positive, but in most instances, it is not.

CT Scan-directed Needle Biopsy

The second way in which a more definitive assessment of the lymph node status can be made is by performing a CT scan-directed aspiration biopsy. This is a less invasive way to sample the abnormal lymph node tissue detected on the CT scan. A radiologist who specializes in performing and interpreting CT scans identifies the abnormalities on the CT scan and then aims a specialized needle at the enlarged lymph nodes, making sure not to hit any vital organs or structures. The needle is attached to a syringe that allows suction to be applied. Once properly placed, the needle's suction is applied and cells from the lymph node flow into the syringe. These cells are then put onto a glass slide, processed, and "read" by either a general pathologist or a cytopathologist.

I would strongly argue that if this type of evaluation is going to be done, it is imperative that both the radiologist and pathologist have experience in doing the procedure and interpreting the specimen. Otherwise, it makes little sense to undergo such an exam if the needle is not accurately placed, or the specimen cannot be read with an expert's eye. There has been concern that if there are cancerous cells in the lymph node, that the needle might "seed" them along its track as it is withdrawn. This is more of a theoretical than a practical possibility. However, on very rare occasions it has happened.

The advantages of this type of approach are clear. If the pathologist's reading is positive for cancer cells, the patient has avoided the operation which was required in the sampling of the lymph nodes as part of a planned radical prostatectomy. When performed well, valuable information is obtained with minimal discomfort to the patient, and alternative treatment programs can be offered. If the biopsy is negative, the patient can be considered for a curative radical prostatectomy (or curative radiation therapy), since the enlarged lymph node seen on CT scan was found not to contain cancer. However, you must also realize that this type of procedure is not 100 percent accurate. The negative result on aspiration biopsy may be contradicted by later testing, especially if you are going for a radical prostatectomy, when the more definite lymph node sampling may also be done.

In other words, an aspiration biopsy is very helpful in examining the treatment options if it is positive, but negative results cannot be absolutely relied on. For the patient considering treatment with radiation therapy, a negative aspiration biopsy provides reasonable justification that definitive treatment can be undertaken even though the patient will never have the more thorough lymph node sampling done in association with the radical prostatectomy. Because of the importance of knowing the status of the lymph nodes, there are circumstances in which patients who elect treatment with radiation therapy will undergo a surgical procedure to obtain and sample adequate nodal tissue. If negative, the patient then proceeds with the radiation therapy after the operation has healed. (This operation is called a pelvic lymphadenectomy and is the portion of the operation done initially on the patient getting a radical prostatectomy.)

Laparoscopic-directed Biopsy

The third and newest approach to assessing the lymph nodes is a procedure called a laparoscopy or laparoscopic-directed lymph node biopsy. This procedure's advantage is the ability to visualize and biopsy directly the lymph nodes in question, thus adding more certainty to the final evaluation. It also avoids the formal operation required in a pelvic lymphadenectomy. It is probably most appropriate for the patient choosing radiation therapy for whom an aspiration biopsy does not provide definite enough information or is impractical, and a more extensive operation is not desired.

In this procedure, the abdomen is inflated with a gas, usually carbon dioxide, and then a series of small incisions (usually four "stab wounds") are made to allow introduction of a fiberoptic tube and a light source for direct visualization of the abdominal organs and the lymph nodes in question. The view of the abdominal contents is projected onto a monitor, allowing the surgeon to view the area enlarged. Through this mechanism, suspicious areas may be biopsied directly.

The advantages of such a procedure are obvious. In the first place, much smaller incisions are required to get at the suspicious nodes. The biopsy is done under direct visualization, and thus reduces the risks of missing the target associated with CT scan-directed aspiration sampling. The actual amount of tissue is larger than that obtained by the aspiration, and in certain cases, may equal the amount of sample obtained by a full-blown surgical operation. Several studies indicate that the laparoscopic techniques recover nearly 80 percent as much of the lymph nodes as the more invasive surgeries. Although not always true, the confidence with which one ascertains whether the nodes are positive or negative can be correlated with the amount of tissue sampled, so here, more is better.

As with any new surgical procedure, there is a learning curve before the average physician in the community can claim proficiency. Laparoscopy is no different, and the early results of complications testify to this. In some of the early reports of the procedure, a number of complications were reported, including damage to vital blood vessels in the abdomen, damage to the bowel, clotting complications, including blood clots to the lungs, infections, swelling of the lower legs and scrotal sac, and urination problems. Fortunately, the incidence of these complications has lessened with experience.

With any surgical or medical procedure, especially a relatively new one such as laporoscopic biopsy, it is essential for your own health and well-being that you be an informed consumer. First of all, find out about the general risks and complications associated with that procedure. I have tried to give you that information for all the procedures discussed in this book. Then ask the person who is going to do the procedure how many of these procedures he or she has performed, the relative complication rate, the average length of stay in the hospital, and what emergency measures are available if there is some catastrophic and unforeseen complication.

Be wary if your physician is reluctant to give such information. You are not offending him or her, but rather trying to get essential details about the person's level of experience and expertise. To me, a defensive attitude on a physician's part is sufficient reason to seek another opinion or to change health-care providers.

4

INTERPRETING THE TESTS

WHAT PSA TELLS US

Today the PSA screening test is very often the first indicator that cancer may be present in the prostate gland. As explained in Chapter 3, the PSA test does not provide the definitive information needed to make a diagnosis. It must be followed by TRUS, DRE, and other noninvasive procedures, and confirmed by biopsy. However, the usefulness of PSA testing is not confined to that initial screening. Properly interpreted, it can provide additional information to help in staging the cancer and examining the treatment options. After treatment, as discussed in Chapter 11, PSA monitoring is the primary tool for measuring treatment success and for detecting early signs of cancer recurrence.

Refinements of the PSA test are continually emerging to help distinguish the reasons for PSA elevation. For example, PSA is found in the bloodstream in two forms—"free" and "bound." Free PSA is unattached to other substances, while bound PSA is attached to another molecule, a protein. Some evidence suggests that the proportion of "free" PSA is lower in patients with prostate cancer. If so, a laboratory analysis that distinguishes free and bound PSA might give us additional assessment information. This is now being used more widely and is called the PSA II test or Free: Bound PSA test. Also, by looking at the PSA data for men of all ages with normal and abnormal prostates, we attempt to expand the interpretive value of the information provided by the standard PSA test. Rather than considering the PSA level alone as an indicator of health or disease, we can also look at the PSA level in relation to the patient's age, the size of his prostate, and the speed with which the level is increasing over time.

PSA and Age

Normal values for PSA blood level are generally below 4.0 ng/ml, but there is a certain arbitrariness to choosing this or any other cut-off level. (Ng/ml stands for nanograms per milliliter, and a nanogram is a billionth of a gram.) Determining the actual range of "normal" values is of great importance, since medical decisions are usually based upon the so-called "upper limit of normal." We know that the prostate enlarges with age and that an enlarged prostate manufactures more PSA. Therefore, is the normal range normal for all men at all ages? Is a value of 3.5 "equally normal" for a seventy-year-old man with benign prostate enlargement and a man of fifty with no symptoms or signs of BPH?

Let's consider the case of a sixty-five-year-old man, who on a screening PSA test had a result of 4.4. If the physician and laboratory established that the top normal value was 4, then this result of 4.4 is defined as abnormal. Depending upon the plan of action that was discussed before the test was done, this patient may undergo further evaluation with DRE, TRUS, and possibly biopsy. Suppose, however, we widened the reference range of normal values from 0–4 to 0–6.5 in older men over the age of sixty. There would be fewer "abnormal" results requiring further testing and perhaps biopsy. The same PSA of 4.4 is now considered normal for this sixty-five-year-old man. Since he has no symptoms and the DRE is normal, he is told that all is okay, and the physician will see him again in another year for another test. So, the definition of a normal result becomes important.

A different situation may apply for a younger patient. What happens if the established normal reference range is lower for men in their forties? If the normal PSA values for this group are set as 0–2.5, a PSA of 3.8 ng/ml would be considered abnormal in a forty-five-year-old man and additional tests may be necessary for that individual.

Several large studies have now looked at the range of distribution of PSA values according to age in patients who otherwise have no abnormalities referable to the prostate gland. The results show that lower values can be considered normal for younger men, while higher values can be accepted as normal for older men. Table 3 lists the age-specific reference ranges arrived at in one large study done at the Mayo Clinic.

Table 3. Age-Specific Reference Ranges for PSA

Age (yr.)	Serum PSA (ng/ml)
40–49	0.0–2.5
50–59	0.0–3.5
60–69	0.0–4.5
70–79	0.0–6.5

Figure 6 demonstrates how the age-specific reference ranges can be used in helping decide upon a diagnostic course of action. The practical implications are that fewer older men will be evaluated with DRE, ultrasound, or biopsy based on PSA values between 4.0 and 6.5, while more younger men will undergo testing for values between 2.5

Figure 6

WHAT IS A NORMAL PSA?

- "Normal values" for PSA

    Consider normal value up to 4

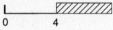

    0   4

- Age specific reference range

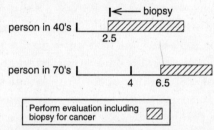

and 4.0. This is an attempt to decrease the number of biopsies in older patients where an elevated value is more likely to be associated with benign enlargement of the prostate gland. Conversely, the practice of using age-specific reference ranges in younger patients is more likely to increase the number of patients found to have abnormal PSA values requiring further testing.

As these age-specific reference ranges are being used in everyday practice, several benefits have resulted. More "clinically important" cancers are being detected and treated in the younger age group of forty to fifty-nine years that would have been missed if the PSA cutoff of 4.0 was used. It has been estimated that nearly three times as many men under age sixty will be considered to have abnormal values when the new reference ranges are used by most or all practitioners. Since these patients have a longer life expectancy, it is desirable to detect and treat their prostate cancers early.

Similarly, fewer invasive tests will be performed in men

over the age of sixty, and the results of some studies suggest that fewer "clinically insignificant" will be treated. In one study, there was a substantial decrease in the number of ultrasound tests and biopsies performed in the over-sixty population when these new age-specific values were used. Since nothing is completely black and white in medicine, there are going to be instances where a potentially important cancer is missed based upon the higher PSA reference ranges. It has been estimated that up to 5 percent of clinically significant cancers may be missed. That figure has to be balanced against the potential for greater suffering from performing many more biopsies. The critical issue in any screening program becomes one of selecting the patients who need to be treated and distinguishing them from those who are better off without or don't need treatment. The age-specific reference ranges seems to be a step in that direction.

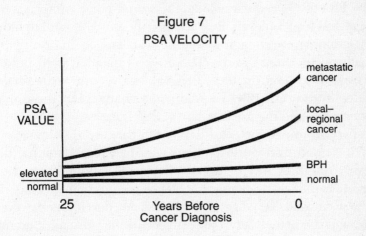

Figure 7
PSA VELOCITY

PSA Velocity

A patient's PSA value can be elevated within the "normal" range. For example, suppose a patient has a PSA value of 1.7 ng/ml and a repeat test a year later indicates a value of 3.6 ng/ml. Both of these values are within the normal limits

KVGC   KALAMAZOO VALLEY
       COMMUNITY COLLEGE
       LIBRARY

but may cause some concern because the value has more than doubled. Should this be a reason for concern, and how should these values, or more importantly the patient, be managed? The rate of change of PSA over time is called the PSA velocity (Figure 7).

The rate at which PSA changes over time might provide important insights into the behavior of the prostate gland, and of any prostate cancer. Could the rate at which PSA changes indicate a lurking cancer or distinguish benign enlargement from cancerous development? In one study done in Maryland, a group of "normal" men were followed for years with periodic physical examinations of their prostate gland and storage of their blood specimens, which permitted future testing. Over a period of some twenty to twenty-five years, some remained well, others developed and were treated for BPH, and a third group were diagnosed and treated for prostate cancer. When the PSA test became available, the stored blood samples were analyzed for PSA levels. Remarkably, the study showed that the PSA values were changing over the years and could distinguish each of the three groups. Those who remained well showed very little change in their PSA values over the years of the study; those with BPH showed some change; but those with cancer showed the greatest rate of PSA increases.

In those patients who developed cancer, the changes in PSA helped distinguish patients who had local/regional disease from those with metastatic disease! Current thinking now suggests that yearly changes of PSA of greater than 0.75 ng/ml per year may be suggestive of cancer development, even though the actual values may still be in the normal reference ranges.

The potential importance of PSA velocity is all too well illustrated by the situation of Kevin Loftus, a fifty-two-year-old university administrator. His PSA level kept doubling every year for four years, but was still well within what is considered the normal range. Finally, Mr. Loftus' PSA level rose from 4 ng/ml to 8 ng/ml, a distinctly abnormal value. Another six months went by before a biopsy was done, demonstrating cancer. He underwent surgery, but the cancer was too extensive to be operable.

Rapid increases in PSA need to be followed up with other diagnostic procedures, but they do not always indicate cancer. Mr. Ted Kazarian, a sixty-nine-year-old professional, had a screening PSA value of 4.7. A DRE was normal. A repeat PSA test done a year later was 9.2. This repeat value prompted a TRUS, which showed some minimally suspicious areas. Based on the rise of the PSA from 4.7 to 9.2, a biopsy was performed and revealed areas of benign enlargement. There was concern, though, because of the near doubling of the PSA over the one-year time frame. Four months later, the value was 9.7, which again prompted a second biopsy. Again the results were negative.

There are several interesting points about this case. It first demonstrates that an elevated PSA is not always indicative of cancer, even with a value in the range of 9–10 ng/ml. The second is the rate of rise of the PSA, in this case from 4.7 to greater than 9. While this is suggestive of a cancer, it does not always mean cancer. The third relates to repeated biopsies. The likelihood of picking up a cancer on the first biopsy series is about 70 to 80 percent. The likelihood goes up to about 95 percent upon second biopsy series. In the case of Mr. Kazarian, if cancer was present and causing the rise of PSA, we would have had a 95 percent chance of diagnosing it with two consecutive biopsies. Furthermore, if cancer was present but undetected despite the biopsies, the likelihood of its being significant is quite low, since the prostate gland had undergone extensive sampling during the two biopsies, with six to eight cores of tissue removed in each biopsy. With this number of samples, the odds of detecting an extensive cancer, if present, are quite high. It is also important to biopsy the transition zone, which is also a likely place for cancer to be found.

PSA Density

A bigger gland will in most cases produce more PSA, so it becomes important to determine whether BPH accounts for all or part of an elevated PSA level. Many men with an elevated PSA have only BPH, while some may have both BPH and cancer. Cancerous prostate cells generally manufacture more PSA per cell than normal cells, so a ratio of PSA level to prostate gland size can help in interpreting whether BPH alone might account for the increased PSA production. The size or volume of the gland can be estimated using TRUS. Dividing the PSA value by the prostate gland volume gives us the PSA density.

If, for example, the serum PSA level is elevated and the volume of the prostate gland is small, the ratio of these two numbers will be higher compared to the same serum PSA value in the presence of a much larger volume gland. Since prostate cancer tissue makes more PSA than normal prostate tissue, we assume that the elevated PSA found in a man with a small gland may be more likely to be due to cancer. When such calculations are performed, a probability of finding cancer can be assigned. A value of 0.15 or greater is suggestive of the presence of cancer, while values of 0.05 are considered to have a low probability of cancer. (See Figure 6 on page 66.) A physician is unlikely to decide whether a biopsy is advisable on the basis of PSA density alone, and many recent studies have cast doubt on its widespread usefulness as a diagnostic tool. Rather, it provides some supplemental information in assessing the significance of the serum PSA test.

PSA and Cancer Staging

While the staging tests described in Chapter 3 provide a clinical stage for the cancer, these tests are often inaccurate in determining the final pathologic or surgical stage, as explained in Chapter 2. In many cases there may be direct extension of the tumor to surrounding tissue (positive margins or extracapsular involvement) or cancerous cells in the lymph nodes that have escaped detection. We cannot know with certainty whether the cancer is organ-confined until the prostate gland and a sample of pelvic lymph nodes are removed surgically and examined by the pathologist. For patients with localized prostate cancer who are treated with radiotherapy, this surgical staging information is often never obtained. It is especially difficult to determine whether the cancer may have extended to involve structures outside the prostate. (Lymph-node status information can be obtained if a separate surgical procedure is done.)

In some circumstances, the PSA test can be used in conjunction with the other diagnostic tests to provide additional preoperative information that can improve our accuracy in determining the staging.

When a prostate cancer sheds cells that find their way to the lymph nodes, bone, or other tissues, these metastasized cells continue to produce PSA that reaches the bloodstream. Very elevated PSA levels suggest more advanced disease—not only a bigger tumor within the prostate, but a higher probability of metastatic disease. While a PSA level below 10 does not rule out the possibility of stage D disease, it would be unusual to find a PSA value as low as, say, 7.5 ng/ml in a patient who has biopsy-confirmed prostate cancer (well or moderately differentiated) and a positive bone scan. Although possible, this scenario is so unusual that some institutions no longer recommend getting a bone scan if the PSA is less than 10 ng/ml at the time of the diagnosis. (I do not agree with this policy.)

In contrast, a patient with a PSA value over 200 ng/ml is unlikely to have localized prostate cancer. He has a high chance of demonstrating X-ray or bone-scan evidence of metastatic spread outside the confines of the prostate gland. Two of my patients represent the range of possibilities, and help to illustrate what PSA does and does not tell us about the extent of the cancer.

Viktor Gabler, a sixty-one-year-old European business-man, came to his doctor with fevers and urinary symptoms that eventually led to an evaluation and biopsy of his prostate gland, which revealed cancer. Mr. Gabler delayed treatment for two years, while he consulted different physi-cians and received different advice, including "wait and see."

Mr. Gabler's father had developed widespread metastat-ic prostate cancer, necessitating bilateral orchiectomy (re-moval of the testicles. This is a procedure used to decrease the amount of male hormones called androgens. Androgens are known to stimulate the growth of prostate cancer. Estro-gens are female hormones that counteract the male hor-mones. Both orchiectomy and estrogens have been used as treatments for metastatic prostate cancer) and estrogen treatments, which could not prevent his death. I cannot help thinking that this nightmarish memory influenced Mr. Gabler in denying the need for treatment. Reassurance that the same fate was not likely to befall him was important in per-suading him to initiate appropriate treatments. Also, the be-lief of many European physicians that prostate cancer often does not require any urgent or curative treatment may have contributed to the delay.

When evaluated at our center, Mr. Gabler had a PSA of 7.6 ng/ml. An asymmetrical gland was seen on transrectal ul-trasound, and a TRUS-guided biopsy revealed Gleason 3 + 2 cancer.

A bone scan was initially read as showing several "hot spots" in the vertebral bodies, ribs, and bones of the neck (the cervical spine). A number of these abnormalities on the scans and X-ray films were thought to be due to arthritis, yet there was one hot spot on the rib that could not be easily explained away. Had the PSA been over a value of 40 ng/ml, there would have been good reason to believe that the rib abnormality was probably a metastasis. The low PSA value argued against performing a biopsy of the rib to determine whether it was cancerous. Based upon Mr. Gabler's clinical stage, Gleason pattern score, and PSA value, we could assign a low probability that the abnormality on bone scan was due to cancer, and were able to spare him an invasive rib biopsy procedure.

Given Mr. Gabler's general good health and good chances, he elected to have a radical prostatectomy. The pathology showed a higher Gleason score of 4 + 3, as often happens at the time of surgical staging, when more of the prostate is sampled. However, the extent of the cancer found confirmed our preoperative interpretation that the patient had organ-confined cancer, with a high likelihood of being cured following radical prostatectomy.

Mr. Wilson Orr also illustrates the relevance of PSA to the diagnostic staging. On routine annual physical examination, this sixty-five-year-old actively retired businessman was found to have a PSA value of 200 ng/ml. While a DRE revealed some areas of hardness, the remainder of the physical exam showed no evidence of distant metastatic spread, making him a potentially curable patient. Despite the fact that a bone scan and abdominal pelvic CAT scan evaluations were all interpreted as either normal or within normal limits, the PSA value was considered to be sufficient evidence that his prostate cancer was probably not localized. His physicians decided against surgical or radiation treatment and Mr. Orr was placed on hormonal treatments.

When Mr. Orr sought my opinion, I held a slightly different view. My initial approach would have differed. In a patient without known metastatic disease, it is important to determine the status of the lymph nodes. My approach would have been to sample the lymph nodes, either by performing a laparoscopic lymph node dissection, or by doing a sampling at the time of contemplated radical prostatectomy. An acid phosphatase test is also a reasonable diagnostic choice in this type of case. If elevated, the likelihood of having extracapsular spread of the prostate cancer is much greater and less amenable to surgical removal. With that information in hand, a more rational treatment approach could ensue. If the nodes turned out to be negative for the presence of metastatic cancer, a curative procedure could reasonably be offered. If positive for metastatic disease, the patient becomes a surgically staged stage D-1 patient, where treatment options vary from observation with no active treatment to early intervention with hormonal treatment. Statistically, based on his clinical stage, Gleason grade, and PSA value, the probability curves predicted a 60 percent chance of having lymph node involvement.

In these two examples, the PSA value was a major factor in sparing patients more invasive and risky diagnostic or therapeutic procedures. In Mr. Gabler's case, a rib biopsy was judged unnecessary, while for Mr. Orr, the very elevated PSA led to the diagnosis of metastatic disease and the choice of hormonal treatment. One could argue that in Mr. Orr's case, the choice of hormonal treatment rather than localized treatment (surgery, radiation) was probably justified given his Gleason grade and elevated PSA. My approach was to give Mr. Orr the benefit of the doubt regarding curability. I saw him six months after his initiation of hormonal treatments, at which time his PSA had declined to the 2 to 3 ng/ml range. His prostate gland was markedly smaller with no discrete abnormalities. Because of these findings, a course of radiation treatments was offered with the hope of eradicating the cancer in his gland, adding to the beneficial effects of the early hormonal treatments.

WHAT THE BIOPSY TELLS US

As explained in Chapter 2, a diagnosis of prostate cancer cannot be made until a biopsy has been done and the tissue has been examined under the microscope by the pathologist. You should understand that the diagnostic information provided by this procedure is not always unambiguous, particularly with early-stage cancers.

First of all, a needle biopsy can only take a small sampling of tissue. A large or disseminated tumor is more likely to be sampled; a small focal cancer has a higher likelihood of being missed, even if the biopsy is guided by ultrasound or DRE abnormalities. This is the reason for repeat biopsies for patients such as Ted Kazarian. With two separate series of biopsies, there is a 95 percent certainty that, if present, a "clinically significant" cancer will be detected.

Diagnosis: PIN

Not all abnormal ("atypical") cells are cancerous ones, and no single feature of an abnormal cell or tissue allows us to say, yes, this is cancer. In some cases the pathologist finds a type of abnormal tissue and cell structure know as *prostatic intraepithelial neoplasia* or PIN. At this time, it is not known for certain whether PIN progresses to prostate cancer, though many researchers believe it is a type of precancerous lesion or abnormality—a stage along the way to the development of a malignancy. It is known that PIN coexists with prostate cancer in more than 85 percent of the cases in which it is found. This makes it a "premalignant marker" or predictor of prostate cancer. Whenever the pathologist returns a diagnosis of PIN, there is a significantly increased likelihood of finding cancer in subsequent biopsies, particularly if the PSA is above 4 ng/ml.

Figure 8

BIG CITY UNIVERSITY HOSPITAL
A TEACHING AFFILIATE OF NORTHERN MEDICAL SCHOOL

DEPARTMENT OF PATHOLOGY
123 MAIN STREET
BIG CITY, USA 99999-8888
434-998-0000

PATHOLOGY REPORT   **PHYSICIAN'S COPY**

PATIENT NAME AND ID NUMBER	DATE OF BIRTH	SEX	ACCESS #
JOHN DOE - 887-998-9999	09-25-32	M	S94-22367

DATE OF PROCEDURE	RECEIVED	REPORT DATE	HOSPITAL LOCAL
4-4-94	4-4-94	4-6-94	SURG OPD

PHYSICIAN   **PATHOLOGIST**
DR. JOHN DOGOOD   DR. REEDEM WRIGHT

FINAL PATHOLOGIC DIAGNOSIS (MICROSCOPIC DIAGNOSIS)

<u>SIX PROSTATE NEEDLE BIOPSIES</u> (S94-22367)

1. **LEFT APEX:**
   <u>PROSTATE ADENOCARCINOMA</u>, GLEASON PATTERN 3 + 4, INVOLV-
   ING 40% OF NEEDLE CORE
2. **LEFT MID ZONE:**
   <u>PROSTATE ADENOCARCINOMA</u>, GLEASON PATTERN 4 + 4, INVOLV-
   ING 50% OF NEEDLE CORE
3. **LEFT BASE:**
   ONE MICROSCOPIC FOCUS <u>SUGGESTIVE, BUT NOT DIAGNOSTIC,</u> OF
   PROSTATE ADENOCARCINOMA. PROSTATIC INTRAEPITHELIAL NEO-
   PLASIA IS PRESENT

4. **RIGHT APEX;**
   BENIGN PROSTATIC TISSUE WITH SOME CELLULAR ATYPIA
5. **RIGHT MID ZONE:**
   <u>PROSTATE ADENOCARCINOMA,</u> GLEASON 3 + 3, WITH A CRIBRIFORM
   PATTERN, AND <u>PERINEURAL INVASION</u> PRESENT IN 90% OF THE NEE-
   DLE CORE.
6. **RIGHT BASE:**
   BENIGN PROSTATE TISSUE

PATHOLOGY REPORT   **PHYSICIAN'S COPY**

PATIENT NAME AND ID NUMBER	DATE OF BIRTH	SEX	ACCESS #
JOHN DOE - 887-998-9999	09-25-32	M	S94-22367

DATE OF PROCEDURE	RECEIVED	REPORT DATE	HOSPITAL LOCAL
4-4-94	4-4-94	4-6-94	SURG OPD

CLINICAL DATA: (SUPPLIED BY PHYSICIAN CARING FOR PATIENT) 62 YEAR OLD MALE, WITH ONE YEAR HISTORY OF INCREASING FREQUENCY, AND IMPOTENCE. DIGITAL RECTAL EXAMINATION SUSPICIOUS FOR BILATERAL INDURATION OF GLAND, WITH DISCRETE NODULARITY ON LEFT SIDE. PSA VALUE OF 22 NG/ML. HIGH CLINICAL SUSPICION OF PROSTATE CANCER.

TISSUE SUBMITTED: THE TISSUE IS RECEIVED IN TWO CONTAINERS, WITH PARTITIONS, LABELED AS RIGHT AND LEFT. IN EACH CONTAINER IS A TRIPLE PARTITION, FURTHER LABELED, APEX, MID ZONE AND BASE THERE ARE SIX NEEDLE CORES PRESENT, EACH MEASURING APPROXIMATELY 0.5 CM IN LENGTH.

GROSS DESCRIPTION: EACH CYLINDRICAL NEEDLE CORE HAS A TAN-GRAY APPEARANCE. EACH TISSUE IS IN A SEPARATE PORTION OF THE RESPECTIVE RIGHT AND LEFT CONTAINER, AND IS LABELED AS RIGHT APEX, RIGHT MID ZONE, RIGHT BASE OR LEFT APEX, LEFT MID ZONE OR LEFT BASE.

ADDITIONAL COMMENTS: THE MAJORITY OF THE TISSUE SUBMITTED CONTAINS GLEASON 3 + 3 OR 3 + 4 PROSTATE ADENOCARCINOMA, CONFIRMING THE CLINICAL SUSPICION OF PROSTATE CANCER. THE DEFINITIVE DIAGNOSIS OF CANCER COULD NOT BE CONFIRMED IN THE LEFT BASE SPECIMEN. IF THIS INFORMATION IS GOING TO AID THE CLINICAL MANAGEMENT OF THE PATIENT, WE CAN SEEK ADDITIONAL CUTS OF THE TISSUE OR SEEK ADDITIONAL CONSULTATION IN INTERPRETING THIS PORTION OF THE TISSUE.

SIGNED:

REEDEM WRIGHT, MD

The Pathology Report

The pathology report (Figure 8) is by far the most important piece of information contained within the medical record in a patient who has been diagnosed with prostate cancer. It is important to understand every component of the report. This particular report is one generated after Dr. Dogood performed needle biopsies on Mr. Doe. The portion of the prostate removed during the biopsy procedure (needle cores) is the tissue which has been processed by the pathology department, and has been "read" by the pathologist, Dr. Wright. The terms *apex*, *mid zone*, and *base* refer to the top, middle, and bottom of the prostate, and indicate where the biopsy needle obtained the tissue from. In this particular biopsy procedure, six individual biopsy specimens were obtained.

The top portion contains information relating to the hospital at which the report was generated. Identifying information about the patient, his date of birth, hospital ID number, and key dates of the biopsy procedure are listed in the top portion as well. The *Access Number* is the specimen identifier, and provides the patient's biopsy specimen with a unique number. This number is particularly important, since several biopsies may have been obtained. If a second opinion is requested, it becomes imperative for the second opinion to check the numbers against one another, so the appropriate biopsy is being interpreted.

The *Final Pathologic Diagnosis* (Microscopic Diagnosis) lists the six pieces of the biopsy, and the accompanying portion of the prostate gland from which they were obtained. While this is the ideal situation, it is not often done in this manner. More commonly, a general statement about the findings on the left and right side are provided, and not as much detailed information, as illustrated here, is provided. The pathologist here was able to provide this type of detailed information since the physician specifically identified the locations of tissue within the prostate as he was obtaining them.

Of the six needle biopsies, three contained definite evidence of cancer. These are numbers 1, 2, and 5. Numbers 4 and 6 had normal prostate tissue without cancer, although number 4 had some atypical cells, of uncertain significance. Biopsy number 3 was complex. The pathologist could not definitely make the diagnosis of cancer in this section but raised the strong possibility that cancer may be present. In this particular illustration this is less critical, since the cancer was found in multiple other areas of the prostate gland. However, if this was the only abnormality, as it may have been in the John Konrad case (see page 83), more information and timely follow-up would have been needed.

The other ideal portion of the *Final Pathologic Diagnosis* (Microscopic Diagnosis) is the fact that the Gleason pattern score is provided in every biopsy that contains cancer, and the percent of cancer found in each needle biopsy core is provided. This is important information, since it provides an estimate of the extent of the cancer. The pathologist, too, has provided even more detailed information by providing other descriptive terms about the cancer such as perineural invasion (which means that there are some cancer cells present), and that a particular type of cancer appearance (cribriform) is present. Both of these features have been thought by some to be associated with different behavior of the cancer.

The *Clinical Data* portion of the report is a nice feature. Here, the physician, Dr. Dogood, provide the pathologist with the relevant information of why the biopsy was performed, and what he is looking for. Without this portion the pathologist may not know why the biopsy was performed, or what the relevant clinical history is. This portion helps focus the pathologist into the reasons why the biopsy was performed in the first place.

The *Tissue Submitted* portion is self-explanatory, and indicates what was actually received from the patient. The *Gross Description*, too, further elaborates on the actual physical appearance of the tissue submitted (as opposed to the microscopic appearance).

The *Additional Comments* section provides a link for both the pathologist, Dr. Wright, and the physician, Dr. Dogood, to communicate with one another. Again, remember the case of Mr. Konrad. The additional comments section was either not read or overlooked, and important information and follow-up were not provided in a timely fashion.

Again, this is what I consider to be an ideal pathology report. Unfortunately, many reports do not contain this type of detailed information. However, by being informed about the essentials of the pathology report, you may help yourself by getting the information which is critical in learning as much as possible about your cancer and arriving upon a treatment plan.

Understanding the Pathology Report

After a needle or surgical biopsy has been made, and the tissue delivered to the laboratory, it is carefully described by a pathology technician, who writes the "gross" description for the pathology report. This includes such important identifying information as the container in which the tissue is shipped to the department, how long the various pieces of tissue are, what their color is, whether there is any blood associated with the tissue, as well as how the tissue sample is labeled.

The tissue specimen is then "processed," meaning that the tissue is immersed in alcohol or other chemicals, and then in paraffin wax, and processed into so-called paraffin blocks. At this point, the fragments of tissue are in the form of small rectangular solids that can then be cut into extremely thin sections—so thin as to allow light to shine through them when placed under a microscope. When the tissue sections are made, they are placed on a glass microscope slide and stained with certain chemicals that impart different colors to various parts (organelles) of the cells that make up the tissue.

The stained tissue sections are placed under the microscope and examined by the pathologist—"read" to provide a final pathologic diagnosis. As mentioned previously, it is the pathologist who makes the diagnosis of cancer, and it is the stained tissue sections that allow the diagnosis to be established.

Each pathologist and institution may "read" slightly differently. For example, one pathologist may grade a given biopsy as Gleason 3 + 3, while another may view the same tissue as a Gleason 3 + 4. In most cases, these subtle differences are not significant. In others, they may be of some importance, since treatment decisions are made in part on the basis of the Gleason grade, just as diagnostic decisions are sometimes based on the PSA level. In these cases, it is often advisable to have another pathologist review the slides—not because the first pathologist is believed to be wrong, but because another pair of eyes may help clarify the diagnostic and treatment possibilities.

This situation occurred with Mr. Douglas Fiedler, a sixty-two-year-old, otherwise healthy man. He was followed for several months with the diagnosis of prostatitis, but when his PSA test, which was initially 16 ng/ml, came down to only 11 ng/ml after intense antibiotic treatment, a biopsy was performed. Eight biopsies were taken in a systematic fashion by his urologist, all of which were returned as negative for cancer and indicating only prostatitis. An elevated PSA persisted in the 11–12 range and prompted a second set of biopsies. One of the eight biopsies was read as showing a focus of moderately differentiated cancer. Because of the associated prostatitis, there was some disagreement among the pathologists interpreting the biopsy specimen. One out of the three argued that according to the definitive criteria for cancer, the pathology found in the biopsy was only suggestive, and not diagnostic for cancer. This prompted a fourth review by another experienced pathologist who confirmed the presence of cancer based upon the pathologic reading of the biopsy specimen.

After the "gross description," the second major portion of the pathologic report is the "microscopic diagnosis" section, which is a short, terse statement of the actual diagnosis. A patient with a diagnosis of prostate cancer would have the phrase "adenocarcinoma of the prostate" listed somewhere in the microscopic section of the pathology report. The findings in the microscopic section are commonly typed in capital letters to command attention. A third component of the pathology report, unfortunately often overlooked, is a descriptive account expanding on the microscopic portion of the diagnosis. This section will describe in detail the various features of the tissue in question, and may oftentimes contain the thinking of the pathologist, especially if the final diagnosis was not crystal clear. It may call to the attention of the attending physician (the physician who performed the biopsy in the first place) the need to consider other possible diagnoses or express the lack of definitiveness of the final microscopic diagnosis. It is, in effect, the "fine print" which sometimes communicates the fact that the diagnosis spelled out in capital letters is not so absolutely certain.

Thus, the pathology report is a component of utmost importance of the medical record. It is not something to be skimmed but needs to be studied closely. It should not just be read by the attending physician but should be discussed in some detail by the physician and pathologist. In the end, the pathology report is the single most important piece of diagnostic information in the patient's medical record. How often is this ideal achieved? Unfortunately, all too infrequently. And for the record, usually no harm will result. However, there are infrequent occasions where a conversation between pathologist and physician may mean the difference between curable and incurable, life and death.

Lost Chances for Cure: The Case of John Konrad

John Konrad, a sixty-two-year-old engineer, had symptoms of urinary frequency and nocturia, accompanied by difficulty maintaining an erection and lessened ability to have sexual intercourse. A visit to his primary-care physician revealed on physical examination a nodular prostate gland, a slightly elevated PSA of 7.9 ng/ml, and an otherwise normal evaluation. A referral to a urologist was approved, taking place about six months after the DRE, at which time a prostate biopsy was done. The diagnostic possibilities considered by the urologist, based on the physical examination, did include the possibility of prostate cancer. Mr. Konrad was told that the biopsy was fine, but to return in six months for follow-up and possibly a repeat biopsy.

The actual wording of the pathology report gave a different, less reassuring message than the one communicated to the patient. Remember the three parts of the report described in the preceding section. In Mr. Konrad's report, the microscopic diagnosis was "small focus of atypical glands (see description)." While this sounds benign enough, the "see description" portion revealed a very different interpretation. This third descriptive section of the report details the atypical features, then concludes: *"The histologic features raise the question of well-differentiated adenocarcinoma but are not considered diagnostic"* (emphasis added).

What does this mean? Simply that the biopsy specimen did not contain the requisite pathological features to be called cancer, but contained enough of these features to raise the suspicion of cancer. In other words, the case is not simply black and white. It means that additional evaluations are necessary to study the troubling features that raise the possibility of cancer (well-differentiated adenocarcinoma) being present. It is not known whether the urologist read the pathology report in its entirety, or whether there was any direct communication between the pathologist and the physician about the ambiguous findings.

It is clear that a series of miscommunications, oversights, and errors of omission occurred that greatly reduced Mr. Konrad's chance of receiving care that would maximize the chances of curing him, or at least maximally control his cancer.

1.   Mr. Konrad was never informed that "cancer" might be present. He did not return for a repeat examination at the time initially recommended by the urologist. Whether this was due to the sense of security (and a false one at that) resulting from the initial "benign" biopsy or the patient's own busy schedule is difficult to know. In addition, the patient intermittently visited his primary-care physician, who had also received a copy of the pathology report. This physician continued to obtain periodic PSA evaluations which remained in the 6–7 ng/ml range.

2.   His attending physician (the urologist who performed the biopsy) and his office never contacted the patient when he did not make an appointment for a six-month follow-up. The patient, too, did not return for the appointment. Both are inexcusable. Systems should be in place to follow patients in whom the medical story is still emerging.

3.   The pathologist probably did not speak with the surgeon about the ambiguous findings on the biopsy. Since the diagnosis of a "small focus of atypical glands" is so nonspecific and so common in many of the thousands of prostate gland biopsies which are performed that do not contain cancer, an attitude of indifference develops.

4.   The sequence of events that should have been set

in motion, initiated by the pathologist in a perfect world, would involve a diligent search and investigation to determine whether a cancer is present or not. This can be approached by having the pathologist ask other, and perhaps more experienced, specialists to review pathology slides. (This is not an ego thing, but a mission to try and provide the patient with the best chance of curing his prostate cancer!) It is common for several opinions to be sought in problematic cases (such as that of Douglas Fiedler) where there are no clear-cut answers. The idea is to try to get a consensus concerning whether a cancer is present and what steps should be taken to get at a more definitive answer.

Why is this so critically important? If Mr. Konrad had received the diagnosis of a well-differentiated cancer associated with a suspicious gland on physical examination and a PSA less than 10 in the fall of 1992, all the hallmarks for cure were present if treated properly. This is the patient's window of opportunity to be diagnosed and cured. If this opportunity is wasted or misused, there is a likelihood that the cancer may spread or may change its favorable microscopic appearance, transforming from a well-differentiated cancer to a poorly differentiated one, greatly decreasing a chance of cure.

Whether such transformations occur has been and always will be a subject of intense debate. Some feel that these transformations into more aggressive forms of cancer occur with regular frequency. Others disagree. Patients in whom it occurs end up sitting in my office discussing the treatment options for the management of metastatic disease, rather than being on the golf course or home with their family, feeling blessed that their cancer was caught at an early enough time to be cured.

You may be wondering whether all these "errors of omission" constitute medical malpractice. The answer is, probably not, but this is not the question on which we should focus. The emphasis needs to be placed on the best application of medical tools and knowledge to provide the patient with the greatest likelihood of cure and improved quality of life. I am not definitively stating that had Mr. Konrad been diagnosed and treated at the time of the biopsy, he would be cured of his cancer. As his story unfolds, you will hear that the likelihood of that happening one and one-half years later (when I first met him) is so low as to be only a remote possibility.

Mr. Konrad continued to have urinary symptoms, which increased in severity. Also, his sexual activity was gradually diminishing, but he attributed this to the "normal aging" process. It was his severe nocturia, in which he woke up to urinate nearly every hour at night, that finally caused him to return to his original urologist for a repeat evaluation about a year and a half later. After the DRE, Mr. Konrad could see that the urologist was alarmed as he told him that a repeat biopsy needed to be done. When Mr. Konrad dutifully took out his appointment book, the urologist abruptly told him to put it away, cancel his appointments, and present himself for the biopsy on Monday, three days hence.

The urgency and the concern visible on the urologist's face reflected the fact that the gland had increased in size in a remarkably rapid fashion. Rather than the lumpy nodules which had been present at the time of the previous DRE, the gland was diffusely hardened, and presented a "ridge" which almost did not allow the examiner's finger to feel the topmost portion of the gland. The physician's record stated that the patient did not return for follow-up as suggested following the diagnosis of atypical glands.

The TRUS and PSA blood tests were performed, the former strongly suggesting the presence of a cancer, the latter being in the same range as before (6–7 ng/ml). The biopsy, to no one's surprise, showed poorly differentiated prostatic adenocarcinoma, Gleason 4 + 4, in both the right and left lobes of the gland.

Needless to say, Mr. Konrad now faced a long course

of treatment and an uncertain prognosis. A year and a half earlier he might well have been diagnosed with a well-differentiated, focal cancer, and now the biopsy showed a poorly differentiated, Gleason $4 + 4$, diffuse cancer, with a high risk of metastases. Was such a cancer present in November 1992? Possibly. We will never know.

I have chosen the case of Mr. Konrad, which will be discussed again in the following chapters, because it represents a series of missed opportunities based upon biases, perhaps ignorance, economic considerations, and poor communication, which collectively taken together constitute marginal medical care. And this type of medical practice is becoming more commonplace with the pressure to control utilization, creating a risk that patients may lose their window of opportunity for cure.

What should you do to ensure that these lost chances for cure do not happen to you? You can certainly ask for a copy of your pathology report, along with other test results. Unless you have a background in medicine or biology, it is unrealistic to expect that you will be able to interpret your own pathology report. Instead, I think the lesson to be learned from Mr. Konrad's experience is the need to probe and to ask questions, to fight your own temptation to accept good news at face value. If you take a passive role, there is a great likelihood that the "system" will fail you in some manner, which in the end could be one of the costliest failures of your life. The lack of communication among the physicians, the pressure to "manage utilization" (limit the number of diagnostic tests and consults), and Mr. Konrad's own willingness to ignore his symptoms all conspired against his receiving appropriate and timely medical attention.

5

Hormones and the Prostate

Thanks to studies done in the early 1940s by Dr. Charles Huggins at the University of Chicago, it has long been known that the male hormones (androgens) have a role in promoting the growth of the prostate and of prostate cancer. Reducing or eliminating the amount of male hormone circulating in the body has a real and substantial impact in shrinking the gland, the primary tumor, and any metastases.

Since Dr. Huggins demonstrated the role of androgens in promoting cancer growth, a discovery that earned him a Nobel prize, hormonal therapies that suppress the body's production of androgens have been a mainstay of the disease's treatment. At this time, hormonal treatment is a standard treatment only for patients with stage C or stage D disease—cancer that is either regionally advanced beyond the prostate capsule or frankly metastatic. However, bold new initiatives now taking place in prostate cancer research suggest that hormonal treatments can benefit patients with localized cancers prior to definitive treatments with either radical prostatectomy or radiation treatments. Additionally, other types of hormonal agents, the 5-alpha reductase inhibitors, are now being studied for use as a preventative in thousands of men who may potentially get prostate cancer later in life.

It is possible that within the next few years, every man with prostate cancer will enter into a conversation with his physician about using hormones for some period of time earlier in the treatment. These drugs, their side effects, and their usefulness in treating prostate cancer are very important to understand.

THE ACTION OF HORMONES ON THE PROSTATE

Testosterone, the most well known of the male hormones, has many complex functions in both males and females. It is not testosterone itself but a metabolite called dihydrotestosterone (DHT) that influences the growth of prostate tissue, including cancer. Testosterone is synthesized primarily in the testes, in response to chemical signals originating in a portion of the brain called the hypothalamus. The hypothalamus signals the pituitary gland, which responds by secreting into the bloodstream another set of chemical signals. One of these signals in turn stimulates the testes to produce testosterone. Other androgens closely related to testosterone are produced in the adrenal glands but in much smaller quantities.

Basically, a hormone is a chemical released by one organ of the body that influences the functioning of another organ, so the chemical signals of the hypothalamus and the pituitary are also hormones, as shown in Figure 9. The hormone released by the pituitary to stimulate the testes to produce testosterone is called *luteinizing hormone*. The hormone secreted by the hypothalamus that is responsible for stimulating the release of luteinizing hormone is called, logically enough, *luteinizing hormone-releasing hormone,* or LHRH. Hormones have important roles in regulating most bodily processes, serving as a sophisticated chemical feedback system. Testosterone and the other androgens are vital to the development of masculine characteristics and to sexual and reproductive functioning. Estrogens and other female hormones perform parallel roles in females. Not so well known is the fact that men also have a certain level of female hormones, and women also have male hormones.

Figure 9

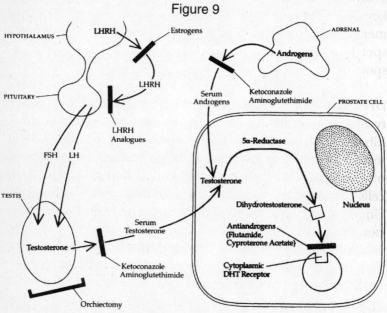

Scheme of achieving castrate androgen levels. Estrogens such as diethylstilbestrol inhibit the release of luteinizing hormone-releasing hormone *(LHRH)* from the hypothalamus, thus also diminishing the release of follicle-stimulating hormone *(FSH)* and luteinizing hormone *(LH)* from the anterior pituitary gland. Analogs of LHRH initially stimulate but ultimately inhibit the release of FSH and LH from the anterior pituitary gland. Ketoconazole and aminogluthethimide inhibit steroid synthetic pathways. In the prostate cells, testosterone is converted into dihydrotestosterone *(DHT)* by the enzyme 5-alpha-reductase. Anti-androgens block the binding of DHT to its cytoplasmic receptor. (Garnick MB. Urologic Cancer. In: Rubenstein E, Federman DD; eds. *Scientific American Medicine.* New York, Scientific American. Section 12, IX:1-17, with permission.)

After it is secreted by the testes, testosterone is metabolized into DHT, its active form. Hormones act on their target tissue by binding to receptors—specialized molecules on the surface or inside of cells that serve to recognize such chemical signals. Each receptor molecule is shaped so that only a specific messenger molecule (or a drug that mimics its shape) can fit "inside" the receptor—an arrangement that is generally compared to a lock (the receptor molecule) and key (the messenger molecule). When a hormone or other messenger molecule "occupies" a cell receptor, it triggers a specific response inside the cell, altering its behavior in response to the signal.

In the case of the prostate cell and its androgen receptors, DHT apparently acts to stimulate protein production, which results in cell division and growth. DHT also appears to inhibit programmed cell death, discussed in Chapter 2, and this may actually be its most important contribution to the growth of the tumor. Cancers grow so rapidly in part because their cells are much less likely to undergo programmed cell death. Under DHT's influence, cell growth increases, even fewer cancer cells die, and the tumor increases in size more rapidly.

THE BASIC STRATEGY

Any treatment that reduces the level of male hormones is called "hormonal therapy." Some of these treatments use hormones or drugs that mimic hormones to interfere with the cycle of testosterone production, while others do not involve the use of hormones at all. The early therapies used surgical castration (an orchiectomy) or a female hormone (DES) to reduce the supply of testosterone to the prostate. The disadvantages of the orchiectomy are obvious, while those of DES were subtle but also significant, as explained in the next section.

As our scientific understanding of the hormonal system advanced, researchers began to look for other, potentially better ways to interfere with the supply of androgen to the prostate. If we look back at Figure 9, we can identify several targets of attack to prevent androgen from reaching its receptor on the prostate gland cells. Would there be any value in combining treatments that aim at different "targets" or use different mechanisms of action? These questions have recently been answered in the positive. Yes, we can devise drugs that interfere at multiple levels of male hormone production and receptor functioning, and that offer advantages in terms of safety and efficacy. The specific drugs now in use are described in more detail in Chapter 13. The process of investigation and discovery (a very exciting process for those who were involved in it) is detailed in the rest of the chapter.

Following Dr. Huggins' discoveries, the early results of hormone-based therapies were so spectacular that researchers believed they had discovered the cure for prostate cancer. This, unfortunately, did not prove true with longer experience. But hormonal treatments are able to diminish the size of the tumor and any metastases quite dramatically, and to slow its growth, often for many years. Eventually, however, the cancer becomes resistant or "refractory" to hormonal treatment.

How this occurs is not completely clear. A prostate cancer-cell colony consists of different types of cells, some of them androgen-sensitive (responding to or requiring DHT) and some adrogen-insensitive (not requiring DHT). The hormonal treatments eliminate or suppress the androgen-sensitive cells, but over time, the androgen-independent cells continue to grow and to resist programmed cell death, until they dominate. It may also be that the receptors change their functioning or configuration in response to the prolonged lack of DHT.

Because the development of hormonally refractory disease appears to be inevitable, hormonal therapy is considered "palliative" rather than "curative." A palliative therapy is one intended to relieve symptoms rather than cure the disease. However, it is important to understand that some individuals with metastatic disease achieve many years of mostly symptom-free life with hormonal treatment, so that the distinction between palliative and curative is not that significant in these cases. Also, some men with localized cancer who receive a course of hormonal treatments followed by surgery have no evidence of cancer when their gland is biopsied. It is not clear why a few men can live many years, even a normal life span, in the presence of metastatic disease, but early treatment and a tumor that is especially sensitive to hormones would seem to be big factors.

WHAT WE HAVE LEARNED AND HOW WE LEARNED IT

At this moment in your life, when you are concerned for your future and your quality of life, you may not be all that interested in history. Yet if hormonal treatments are recommended to you, this information can help you evaluate and understand the therapy offered. Many men are still being offered our two oldest forms of hormonal therapy, surgical castration and the female hormone DES, even though safer and more tolerable therapies are now available.

The VA Studies—Round One

When I was a medical student nearly twenty-five years ago, prostate cancer was commonly diagnosed in an elderly man who had significant or severe problems with urination. More often than not, the patient would already have metastatic disease at the time the cancer was diagnosed. Many patients, in fact, were first diagnosed when the bone metastases resulted in crippling pain or fracture. After emergency treatment for the presenting problem, these men would be given hormonal therapy.

The removal of male hormones in these stage D patients resulted in very substantial benefits. The cancerous involvement in the bones would diminish in size, as shown on the X-rays, and there would often be a dramatic decrease in bone pain caused by prostate cancer. Some patients experienced miraculous relief of bone pain within hours of decreasing the levels of male hormones. So dramatic, in fact, was the relief afforded by this treatment that many thought that the disease was actually being cured by such treatment.

At that time, there were two basic approaches to eliminating the male hormones. The first was to administer the female hormone known as DES (diethylstilbestrol), which inhibits the production of LHRH by the hypothalamus. As a result, testosterone production by the testes is suppressed. The second, more radical approach, was to remove the testes in a surgical procedure called bilateral orchiectomy. This surgical procedure was relatively safe, since it had only limited risks associated with the use of anesthesia and the possibility of postoperative infection. But the psychological stress could be very severe, especially when there were few emotional support systems available to help the patient cope with his changed body image.

The side effects associated with DES took more time and study to determine. A series of studies undertaken by the Veterans Administration (VA) in the late fifties and early sixties provided important information on the value of DES treatment, as well as many other issues in the management of all forms of prostate cancer. These studies are well worth reading about. Many physicians who went through medical school in the seventies or later only know about the VA studies secondhand, or not at all.

The first VA study compared four treatments for prostate cancer: 1. DES high dose (5 mg/day); 2. orchiectomy alone; 3. orchiectomy plus DES (5 mg); and 4. placebo (no treatment). This study design served to address the logical first question: Was the combination of surgical castration and DES better then either modality alone?

The VA study showed no advantage to the combination of DES and orchiectomy. Those who were treated with the high dose of DES did benefit in terms of apparently slowed progression of their disease. However, these mostly elderly men had a much higher death rate from heart attack and other cardiovascular disease. Any benefit in terms of cancer was wiped out by the increased risk of heart disease.

These results were completely unexpected. At the time, it was believed that female hormones might protect the body against heart disease, since women have a lower incidence of heart attack than men. At the same time that the VA studies were taking place, the National Heart and Blood Institute was studying whether taking DES might reduce the incidence of heart attack for men who were at high risk. These men turned out to have a higher incidence of heart disease with DES than without it! So the enthusiasm for DES as a treatment for all men and for all stages of prostate cancer came under serious attack.

The second startling finding from these initial VA studies had more profound implications for the overall treatment of prostate cancer. Prior to the study, it was accepted that hormonal treatment for prostate cancer was associated with a prolonged survival. When the data from these studies was analyzed, the researchers were unable to find any survival benefit in patients with stage C or stage D disease.

Additional studies were designed and conducted by the Veterans Administration. The results of these studies unequivocally confirmed the major findings in the initial study—that DES in certain higher doses caused excessive cardiovascular side effects, and that overall survival was not improved due to this increased incidence of cardiovascular disease, even though patients may have had a slowing of prostate cancer progression.

These studies formed the foundation for the management of metastatic prostate cancer until recently. Because prolonged survival had not been demonstrated and the major benefit of hormonal therapy seemed to be relieving pain and urinary symptoms, the use of hormones was redefined as a palliative treatment—that is, a treatment that could not cure the disease, but could alleviate the patient's symptoms, if and when they occurred.

The VA Studies—Round Two

The second major VA investigation tried to determine the optimal dose of DES for use as a palliative treatment. The idea was to analyze the incidence of side effects with DES at different doses, to see if one dose might maximize the therapeutic benefits while minimizing the incidence of cardiovascular complications. Stage C and D patients were randomly assigned to receive one of four treatments: 1. DES at a dose of 5 mg/day; 2. DES at a dose of 1 mg/day; 3. DES at a very low dose of 0.2 mg/day; or 4. placebo (no treatment until symptoms developed).

As in the first study, patients exposed to the highest dose of DES again demonstrated a higher rate of cardiovascular side effects. This complication caused premature closure of the study, because the 1 mg dose of DES seemed to provide all of the anticancer benefits, with a lower risk of side effects. When the analysis was completed, it appeared that the DES-treated patients had little advantage in terms of overall survival compared to the placebo-treated patients. In reality, the patients who were randomly assigned to receive placebo received no treatment only until they developed symptoms that required some sort of treatment. A more appropriate term for this group of patients would have been "delayed hormonal treatment." It became commonly accepted as fact, based in large part on the results of these studies, that hormonal treatments probably do not increase survival; that if hormonal treatment was to be utilized, it was probably best initiated when the patients developed symptoms, since the treatment was in fact palliative rather than curative in nature.

The VA Studies Revisited

Then, in 1987, the National Institutes of Health convened a conference to develop a consensus on the management of localized prostate cancer—what the various treatments should be, who should receive such treatments, what were the side effects of treatment, and what future directions in prostate cancer research should be pursued.

As a part of that conference, all the data from the Veterans Administration studies were updated and reanalyzed. A very important finding emerged. In all of the previous statistical analyses of the VA data, patient outcomes were analyzed according to specific stage of disease. Patients with stage C or D disease receiving any of the four treatments did not show any significant increase in survival time.

The senior biostatistician (the late Dr. David Byar) tried something different when he reanalyzed the second VA study. Instead of separating patients into the stage C and D categories, he combined the two groups. By doing so, it turned out that there was indeed an improvement in the survival of patients who were treated with hormonal therapy compared to those who did not receive treatment, or who were treated at a later time point in their disease.

This reanalysis had profound implications. Could survival for men with advanced prostate cancer (stage C and D disease) be improved if hormonal treatment was started early on, rather than reserving the treatments for patients who developed symptoms that needed to be controlled or palliated?

Based upon the VA studies, the recommended treatment for patients with either stage C or stage D prostate cancer was to administer DES at a dose of 1 milligram. This dosage was found to maximize the anticancer activity but minimize the side-effect profile that accompanied the 5 mg dosage DES. The 0.2 mg dosage was found to be the same as placebo. A series of subsequent investigations found that the 1 mg dosage of DES could not consistently maintain "castrate levels" of testosterone. In other words, even though this dose of DES initially knocked down the levels of testosterone and DHT to the same as a surgical castration, which eliminates 95 percent of the circulating androgens, over time the levels usually crept back up, so a substantial number of patients "escaped" from the therapeutic action of the hormone. Nearly every important study since that time has studied the effects of DES at a dosage between 1 and 5 milligrams. The clinical dosage most commonly used was established at 3 mg.

Significant cardiovascular effects still occurred at 3 mg. Although not as severe as at the 5 mg dosage, heart attacks, pulmonary blood clots, and the development of congestive heart failure continued to be reported, raising concern about the overall utility of DES.

The LHRH Analogues

In the mid 1980s, researchers from both academia and industry were working on the development of a new class of drugs to attempt to achieve the same benefit as DES and orchiectomy, but without the cardiovascular side effects of the drug or the psychological impact of a castration. The idea was that interrupting the pathways by which male hormones are produced and released could provide an effect similar to removal of the testicles.

I and my colleagues, Dr. Michael Glode from the University of Colorado, Dr. Jay Smith then at the University of

Utah, and Drs. Devorah Max and John Seely from TAP Pharmaceuticals, did the initial clinical work in the development of a new class of drugs called LHRH analogues. We first conducted studies designed to determine the effectiveness and dosing, and then did a pivotal study comparing the new drug leuprolide to DES. We showed that the efficacy of leuprolide was comparable to DES, yet it was without the severe cardiovascular side effects. These studies served as a basis for FDA approval of the first LHRH analogue for the treatment of metastatic prostate cancer.

The term *LHRH analogue* means that these compounds are chemically similar to the hormone released by the hypothalamus to begin the cycle of testosterone synthesis. The LHRH analogues interfere with the delicately balanced chemical feedback system that stimulates and controls testosterone production in the testes. After causing a brief surge of testosterone synthesis, their continued administration results in a shutdown of the synthesis of the hormones from the hypothalamus and the pituitary that control production of testosterone in the testes. The effect of administering these drugs mimics the surgical procedure of removing the testes—the main source of androgens. Remarkably, these medicines are devoid of major side effects, except for eliminating sexual interest and potency, a side effect of all the long-term hormonal therapies and the testosterone "flare" caused by the brief initial surge.

The Antiandrogens

The early and mid 1980s also saw research into another class of compounds known as the *antiandrogens*. As seen in Figure 9, this class of drugs is able to interfere with the interaction of DHT with its receptor in the prostate cancer cell. The antiandrogens preferentially occupy the receptor, displacing DHT and preventing it from stimulating the cells to grow and divide. However, feedback mechanisms signal a shortage of testosterone/DHT reaching the cells and result in increased production of testosterone, some of which will still reach and occupy the receptors.

The prototype antiandrogen used in the United States is called flutamide (Eulexin) and was developed by Schering-Plough Corporation. Early studies of its efficacy as a single treatment produced good results, but the investigational drug did not receive much "press" as a new and urgently needed treatment. That all changed when a Canadian physician named Dr. Ferdinand Labrie started making some important claims of success in treating metastatic prostate cancer with combination programs that included an antiandrogen.

Combination Hormonal Treatment

The scientific hypothesis Dr. Labrie posed was whether prostate cancer patients could enjoy better cancer control and cancer-cell killing if two hormonal agents, each with a distinct mechanism of action, were used together. Since nearly 95 percent of circulating levels of androgens originate from the testes, most treatments had focused on eliminating testosterone supplied by the testes, either medically using DES or an LHRH analog, or surgically with a bilateral or-chiectomy. However, what about the 5 percent of circulating levels of androgens produced in the adrenal glands? (The adrenal glands, mentioned in Chapter 2, are two small glands located above the kidneys which synthesize a variety of hormones, including adrenaline, steroids, and androgens.)

Labrie theorized that this small amount of male hormones could be important in continuing to fuel the growth of prostate cancer cells. Drawing on reasonably good experimental evidence, he argued that the prostate cancer growth was exquisitely sensitive to even minute amounts of male hormones. An antiandrogen could prevent these small amounts of androgens from exerting their influence on cancer cell growth. Combined with the use of an LHRH analogue to halt testosterone production in the testes, antiandrogens had the theoretical possibility of having a stronger anticancer effect.

The debate over the next few years centered as much on the egos of the researchers and authorities involved as it did on the scientific merits of Labrie's theory. Labrie was charged with inappropriately selecting patients who had the best or most favorable type of cancers, patients who were going to do well regardless of what type of treatment was going to be used. Scientific investigations involving animals did not seem to support Dr. Labrie's theory. But it was rapidly becoming a battle of personalities rather than evidence.

In the meantime, patients desperate for treatment for their metastatic disease were flocking to the Labrie clinic in Quebec. To obtain the investigational antiandrogen in the United States, the patient's physician had to go through extensive regulatory red tape. It was easier for the patient to go to Quebec to obtain the antiandrogens, bring them back into this country, and take them with or without the knowledge of his local physician. While this turned out to be a practical solution for those with the means to travel to Canada and pay for the expensive treatments, it was not so for the majority of patients.

Dr. Vincent DeVita, then the Director of the National Cancer Institute (NCI), initiated a study under the direction of Drs. David Crawford and Mario Eisenberger and David McLeod to help resolve the issues and provide guidance for patients and physicians alike. Dr. DeVita addressed the most basic question: Does the use of an antiandrogen, such as flutamide, when added to an LHRH analogue, such as leuprolide, provide any benefit to the management of patients with metastatic prostate cancer?

This study randomly assigned 600 volunteers to receive one of two treatments: either the LHRH analogue leuprolide plus a placebo, or leuprolide plus the antiandrogen flutamide. The 600 patients enrolled in the study included those with different degrees of metastatic disease (minimal to extensive "tumor burdens" as measured by bone and CT scan) and differing levels of functional impairment, from those who were fully active to those who were bedridden. Tumor burden refers to the amount of cancer a patient has, usually determined by measuring the cancerous deposits seen on bone scan or other scans. A few abnormal spots would be considered "low" tumor burden. Many abnormal spots, or cancer deposits in areas other than bone, would signify a "high" tumor burden. The tumor burden was determined for these patients and they were each assigned a functional performance status using a standard scale. The study was designed to determine whether the addition of the antiandrogen increased survival time in patients with metastatic disease, or whether the quality and duration of the therapeutic response might be improved.

Overall, this important study showed a greater than seven-month survival advantage for the group who received the combination treatment of the LHRH analogue and the antiandrogen. However, the patients with a low tumor burden and a good performance status showed the greatest benefit, with a nearly two-year survival advantage. The finding of a better outcome with the combination treatment for all patients and a significant improvement in the minimal-disease good-performance status patients has profound implications, again supporting early treatment. Along with the reanalysis of the VA studies, the NCI study indicates that hormonal treatment does more than relieve symptoms of metastatic disease, it can also extend survival.

Several other studies have looked at effects of the combination of an antiandrogen with bilateral orchiectomy, or the addition of an antiandrogen to other LHRH analogues. While not all studies have yielded the same results, several confirmed the findings of the initial NCI study. Based upon the NCI study, the FDA approved the use of flutamide in combination therapy with an LHRH analogue for patients with metastatic prostate cancer (stage D2).

More recent research has suggested that a greater proportion of the body's androgens may be produced in the adrenal glands—an estimated 30 percent of the total, not 5 percent as previously thought. This discovery provides further support for Dr. Labrie's theory about the significance of the adrenal glands' contribution to the supply of androgens reaching the prostate cancer.

Other agents sometimes used in combination hormonal therapy include ketoconazole and aminoglutethimide, which inhibit synthesis of testosterone in the adrenal glands.

Hormonal Prevention?

Studies are now underway to evaluate potential uses for another type of hormonal agent, the 5-alpha reductase inhibitors, represented by finasteride (Proscar). Proscar reduces the levels of DHT in the prostate by blocking the action of 5-alpha reductase, the enzyme that is responsible for converting testosterone to DHT. Proscar is currently approved as a medical treatment for BPH, for which it provides a modest benefit by shrinking the gland and relieving urinary symptoms. Proscar has shown little value as a treatment for prostate cancer, but it is now being studied in a very large seven-year trial, involving 18,000 healthy volunteers, to see if it might have some benefit in preventing prostate cancer.

6

WHO GETS PROSTATE CANCER, AND WHY?

Several patients I treated were convinced that obsessive masturbating as an adolescent was the cause of their prostate cancer, and I could not persuade them that this is not true. Their belief points to the fact that we often hold ourselves responsible for our illnesses, or at the very least, we want to know the answer to the question, "Why me?" In regard to prostate cancer, the answer is not yet clear. We have identified a number of risk factors—some of them genetic, and some of them environmental and possibly preventable. This is information you might want to know to understand your disease a little better, and you may also want to share it with a brother, son, or friend who has some of these risk factors.

There is also some slight evidence to suggest that the modifiable risk factors, particularly dietary ones, could have an impact on the rate at which the cancer advances. This possibility is something you should consider in your self-care. Dr. William Fair has recently shown that dietary modification by decreasing fat intake may be important in decreasing the risk of prostate cancer.

ABOUT RISK FACTORS

There are a number of risk factors associated with prostate cancer. A risk factor is not necessarily a cause, though it often points to one. It can be simply an association, meaning that a significant number of people who get disease x also have characteristic y, but there is no clear cause-and-effect relationship. For example, it has been fairly conclusively proven that smoking causes lung cancer. However, smoking is also a risk factor for a large number of other medical conditions, including bladder cancer. In some cases, smoking may well be a contributing factor to developing the disease. In other cases, it may be simply an association, perhaps meaning that people who smoke are more likely to make other lifestyle choices that put them at risk. Either way, a risk factor serves as an indicator that the individual has a greater chance of developing the condition in question.

FAMILY HISTORY

Prostate cancer runs in families. If your brother, your father, or one of your father's brothers has had prostate cancer, you are more likely to develop it. This fact has been incorporated into the screening programs' recommendations advising men with a positive family history for prostate cancer to begin annual screening at an earlier age.

TESTOSTERONE LEVEL

Because male hormones are known to influence prostate growth, it has been suggested that the long exposure to these hormones may in some way promote eventual development of prostate cancer. Hormone levels vary from individual to individual, and it may be that men with higher levels are at greater risk. Men who lose their testes at an early age rarely, if ever, develop prostate cancer, suggesting that male hormones are necessary for the development of the disease. More research is clearly needed on this subject.

GEOGRAPHY

Recent data has suggested that death rates from prostate cancer vary geographically, with higher rates occurring at northern latitudes in countries such as Iceland, Sweden, Norway, and Switzerland. However, this may be explained by the fact that many European physicians do not generally opt to treat prostate cancer. It has been suggested that exposure to ultraviolet (UV) light may be a protective factor against prostate cancer development. This may be in some way linked to alterations in vitamin D metabolism. If true, this would have important implications for developing preventive strategies.

Other striking geographical differences may be related to culture, lifestyle, and most importantly diet, as discussed in the following sections. Clinically detectable prostate cancer is extremely uncommon in China and Japan. It has been estimated that a black male living in San Francisco is 120 times more likely to develop prostate cancer than a native Chinese male living in China.

RACE, NATIONALITY, AND ETHNICITY

African-Americans have the world's highest incidence of the disease, about twice as high as U.S. whites—and thirty- to fiftyfold greater than native Japanese and Chinese men! The extraordinary racial, ethnic, and national differences in the incidence of prostate cancer are one of the most intriguing clues to unraveling its causes and possible prevention.

You might assume that these enormous racial variations in incidence arise from genetic differences, but environment and lifestyle appear to be of equal significance. For example, although clinical detectable cancer is relatively rare in native Chinese and Japanese men, recent evidence suggests that latent cancer (microscopic disease that is not likely to be detected during an individual's lifetime except by PSA screening) has a similar incidence in Japanese men. (About 15 percent to 30 percent of all men over fifty are estimated to have some cancerous prostate cells, rising to about 60–70 percent of men by age eighty.) What's more, when Japanese men immigrate to the United States and assume an "American" lifestyle, the incidence of clinically diagnosed prostate cancer approaches that of the total U.S. male population. These types of findings point to the presence of some environmental factor that may activate latent cancer into cancer that is more aggressive, and more likely to cause problems and be diagnosed because of symptoms referable to the cancer.

The fact that the risk of prostate cancer is twice as high for U.S. Blacks as for U.S. whites may also be due to either genetic or environmental factors, or both working together. Black men in Africa and Asia are not nearly at as high a risk as U.S. Blacks. We know that African-Americans are more likely to be diagnosed at a later stage of the disease, and the likelihood of a U.S. black man dying from the disease is nearly twice that of his white counterpart. This disparity may well be due to generally poorer access to health care, but some evidence suggests that the cancers that develop in black men are more likely to be aggressive. One study has suggested that college-age Blacks have a slightly higher level of male hormones—both testosterone and DHT—compared to whites of the same age group. Much more needs to be done to understand why African Americans are more likely to develop and to die from prostate cancer—and to use this information for early detection and treatment, or prevention.

VASECTOMIES AND BPH— POSSIBLE BUT NOT PROVEN

Many men have been alarmed by reports that having had a vasectomy increases the risk of later developing prostate cancer. The two studies made of the association between vasectomy and prostate cancer have concluded that men with vasectomies have one-and-one-half times the risk of prostate cancer than men who have not had vasectomies. That may seem like a substantial risk to you, but by comparison heavy smokers have ten to twenty times the risk of developing lung cancer compared to nonsmokers. Vasectomy and prostate cancer are both very common, so a slight association between the two may not be truly meaningful. More research is needed.

Likewise, the association of prostate cancer with benign enlargement of the gland is unclear. BPH is very common— but the theory that it predisposes to the development of cancer is not well supported. Many men do have both BPH and prostate cancer, or are initially diagnosed with BPH and later found to have cancer. As mentioned in Chapter 2, before the development of the PSA blood test, early asymptomatic cancers were most often detected in men treated surgically for BPH with TURP (transurethral resection of the prostate). When the "chips" of prostate tissue removed via TURP were biopsied, they were found to contain microscopic cancer.

However, BPH and cancer generally, not always, occur in different parts of the gland. BPH arises in the inner, transitional zone of the gland, where it causes its characteristic problems by squeezing the part of the urethra that passes through the inner gland. Cancer most often develops first in the peripheral zone adjacent to the rectum. Likewise, there has also been concern that the TURP procedure may increase the risk of later developing prostate cancer, but there is no convincing evidence to support this.

If you now have a diagnosis only of BPH, there is no reason to fear that you are more likely to develop cancer than any other man your age. However, since distinguishing between BPH and cancer can sometimes be difficult with our current diagnostic tests, you would be well advised to learn about the sometimes subtle diagnostic distinctions. PSA density and velocity, discussed in Chapter 4, are helpful concepts to understand. If you are considering being treated for BPH with finasteride (Proscar), you should know that this drug causes the PSA level to drop. This effect of Proscar on PSA may "mask" the elevation in PSA that would normally help us detect a growing cancer. For this reason, it is important to have a "baseline" PSA level measured before beginning treatment with Proscar. There are clinical studies now underway to see if Proscar might have some value in preventing the development of prostate cancer, based on its influence on the availability of DHT to the prostate (see Chapter 5).

DIET AND LIFESTYLE

Diet seems to be the big factor, and may well account for the racial and geographical data. Animal fat is the dietary component that has been implicated most commonly in the development of prostate cancer. In countries in which large amounts of animal fat are consumed (such as our own!), the incidence of prostate cancer is higher. This parallels the increased risk of breast cancer for women residing in countries where large amounts of dietary animal fat are consumed. In contrast, populations of men who ingest large amounts of dietary fiber may actually have a *lower* incidence of prostate cancer. These patterns in dietary fat consumption may well have a role in the national and ethnic differences in prostate cancer incidence already discussed.

The most compelling information relating dietary animal-fat consumption to prostate cancer is the association with death rates. Populations exposed to higher animal-fat consumption have a higher death rate associated with prostate cancer, compared to populations in which the animal-fat consumption is lower. Most of the large studies that have attempted to study this association have shown such differences, although not all have. How the unsaturated animal fat might act to promote prostate cancer development, or induce latent cancer to grow more rapidly, is a topic of intense investigation.

Other factors that have been associated with prostate cancer development include socioeconomic factors, job, smoking, exposure to various industrial toxins such as cadmium, frequency of sexual activity, and a history of prostatitis. There are both positive data, that is, information suggesting that the presence of these factors may predispose to the development of prostate cancer, and negative data, suggesting just the opposite. The best documented risk factors remain family history, race/ethnicity, age, and dietary animal-fat consumption.

The recommendations that now have been endorsed by the American Urological Association and American Cancer Society reflect these factors. African-American men and those with a family history of prostate cancer should be screened annually with PSA and DRE beginning at age forty. Otherwise, men over the age of fifty should be screened with an annual PSA test and DRE.

LIFESTYLE CHANGES CAN'T HURT, MIGHT HELP

It seems clear that diet is probably a very important factor in predisposing men to the development of prostate cancer. Of equal importance, modifications in dietary intake may even prove to be a potential preventive measure which may actually decrease the risk of developing prostate cancer. Very recent studies by Dr. William Fair are now being conducted indicating that a man's PSA test value can decrease if a certain type of low-fat high-fiber diet is adopted! Studies that evaluate dietary factors are likely to continue to be done. Just recently, a diet that included fruit fiber was shown to decrease the aggressive behavior of prostate cancer in an experiment with animals. We will have to continue to wait for additional studies to be performed before definitive answers emerge.

Other diets some believe decrease risk include increased consumption of tomatoes, beans, raisins, and other dried fruit. Other, more skeptical researchers feel that such findings are not well substantiated. In general, however, I cannot argue with the practice of encouraging a high-fiber low-animal-fat diet. Since the overall health benefits of such a diet are well established, it makes good sense to cut your animal fat consumption. You will certainly improve your overall cardiovascular health, and the lifestyle change could conceivably reduce the aggressiveness of microscopic disease.

7

CURRENT TREATMENT OPTIONS FOR LOCALIZED PROSTATE CANCER

This brief chapter outlines the treatment options for localized prostate cancer—stages A, B, and some stage C disease. Chapters 8 through 10 examine these options more thoroughly. My purpose here is to suggest considerations and guidelines that may help you in determining which treatment is most appropriate for you.

When the results of the DRE, TRUS, and other diagnostic procedures suggest that the prostate cancer is curable by localized treatment modalities, the following treatment options are available.

I. The Standard Therapies
    A. Surgery to remove the prostate gland, either:
        1. Radical prostatectomy (either retropubic or perineal), removing the entire gland and neighboring tissues, or
        2. Nerve-sparing prostatectomy (also called "anatomic" prostatectomy), which attempts to preserve nerves and blood vessels (surrounding the prostate gland) needed for an erection
    B. Radiation therapy, to destroy the cancerous cells, either:

1. External-beam radiation therapy, in which the radiation dose is delivered by an external source that targets the cancer as precisely as possible, or

2. Brachytherapy, the insertion of radioactive "seeds" directly into the prostate gland, or

3. Combination therapy—both external beam and brachytherapy

II. Nonstandard or Investigational Therapies
   A. Neoadjuvant therapy followed by radiation or surgery—pretreatment with hormones to shrink the cancer before definitive treatment with radiation or surgery
   B. Cryosurgery—using special probes to subject the gland to extreme cold, killing the tissue

III. Watchful Waiting—No active intervention is offered until the disease progresses.

About "Watchful Waiting"

As I have said, I consider watchful waiting an appropriate choice for a minority of patients—primarily elderly men or those with other serious medical conditions—diagnosed with stage A1 or T1c, well-differentiated (low Gleason grade) focal (not diffuse or disseminated) disease. These are men who might be reasonably expected to "die with" rather than "die of" their prostate cancer, or who might be too frail to tolerate the potential complications of treatment. I do not consider a healthy, active man in his seventies to be "elderly." In presenting the options to these patients, I recommend active intervention rather than playing the odds that either it is a latent or slow-growing cancer, or that we will be able to detect and treat its localized advance before it sheds cells into the bloodstream.

George Parisi represents the type of patient for whom many physicians would recommend no treatment. At the age of seventy-one his PSA value was 7.1 ng/ml, and it rose to 7.4 a year later. A biopsy found a single cluster ("focus") of cancerous cells, while a lymph-node biopsy was negative. After discussion, Mr. Parisi decided that he did want to seek a definitive, early treatment. He had a radical prostatectomy with no significant complications. Although he was moderately sexually active before surgery and did not recover his potency after treatment, a possibility that had been thoroughly discussed, he was very satisfied with his decision and its outcome. One year later his PSA level was still undetectable, a strong indicator that the cancer was eliminated.

In addition to detecting cancer at earlier stages, we are now diagnosing it in younger men. For these men, faced with the prospect that treatment may very well leave them partially or entirely impotent, the advice to opt for watchful waiting can be very attractive. However, to date our data suggest that the type of cancer diagnosed in younger men tends to be more aggressive, making the choice between treatment and nontreatment still more difficult.

If you are advised to take a course of watchful waiting, or if your physician chooses this course for you, be advised that all health-care professionals are under increasing pressure to "control utilization"—to limit the number of costly diagnostic and treatment procedures. Radiation treatments cost $15,000 (conformal 3D radiation treatments about $30,000–$40,000), while the bill for prostate surgery is in the neighborhood of $15,000–$25,000. I am not for the moment suggesting that your physician would deliberately deny you needed treatment to save your insurer money. Rather, the point is that the arguments in favor of nonintervention or delayed intervention are very attractive to health-care policymakers who have the formidable task of controlling our staggering health-care costs.

If you are persuaded to accept a policy of nonintervention or watchful waiting, be certain that your diagnostic work-up and assessment have been as thorough and sophisticated as our current techniques allow, and that your interests and requirements have truly been given priority in the decision.

Evaluating the Treatment Options

The active interventions for localized cancer have been classified here as "standard" and "nonstandard." A nonstandard treatment is not necessarily "experimental." Rather, it is a relatively new therapy with demonstrated short-term efficacy and an acceptable side-effect profile, but for which we do not yet have long-term outcomes. Arguably, by this definition, nerve-sparing prostate surgery and brachytherapy could be considered nonstandard, since they involve recent innovations and advances in techniques for which we do not yet have long-term survival data. The other definition of nonstandard is a treatment that your insurer may not yet routinely approve for reimbursement. In other words, if you choose a nonstandard therapy, you may have a struggle to get the needed okay and referral from your insurer, HMO, or other managed-care organization.

There are risks, complications, and trade-offs for all these options that need to be carefully weighed. No option is ideal for every patient, and choices are usually individualized. Your doctor's responsibility is to assess all your diagnostic information, your age, and your general state of health and to use this information to make treatment recommendations to you.

Ideally, your physician will also have a discussion with you about your quality-of-life expectations and requirements. You may be most concerned about maximizing your chance for a total cure. Or you may opt to accept a higher risk of recurrence five or ten years later in exchange for maximizing your chances of retaining sexual potency. This should be a genuine discussion, in which your physician listens to your concerns and requirements, and in which you also fully understand the risks and implications of the priorities you have set. I have had patients who made "at-all-costs, never-mind-the-consequences" decisions that I considered irrational, and in one instance I had to withdraw from the treatment team when I thought the decision was not good medicine. Nonetheless, I have always considered that only you, the patient, can know your own quality-of-life requirements and that these must always be factored into the treatment choice.

For most men with localized cancer, the basic treatment choice is surgery or radiation. You may well get conflicting views and advice from your physicians, if both a radiation therapist and a surgeon are involved in evaluating your disease. Surgeons, naturally enough, feel that surgery is the treatment of choice for otherwise healthy men with localized cancer. They point to the fact that the five-year survival rate is generally lower for patients treated with radiation therapy. However, *because* surgery is viewed as the treatment of choice for younger men with no other medical conditions, those who receive radiation treatments tend to be older men in poorer health, whose odds for long-term survival should be expected to be lower.

This is a complex issue involving what physicians call patient-selection criteria. Who is the ideal candidate for treatment *x*? The advantages and disadvantages of radiation therapy versus surgery have been endlessly debated and will continue to be debated. You may have certain risk factors that increase the likelihood of complications with one treatment or another. For example, it is certainly the case that an older man in poor health is not a good candidate for surgery.

As you learn about all these treatment options, be careful to weigh the possible complications carefully. While you don't want to focus on the worst possible outcome—for example, the 0.1–0.8 percent mortality rate of prostate surgery—neither should you cross your fingers and trust that you will be one of the lucky ones who have no complications and no side effects.

Reading the following chapters and learning in detail about the various treatment options is essential to making an informed, personal decision about what is best for you. It is equally essential to ask questions and learn about the individuals who will be providing the treatment you choose. Published complication rates average data from different studies and surveys. Surgery is a skill, however, and so is radiation therapy. Some surgeons have complication rates much lower than the published data, and some much higher. Likewise, the expertise of the radiation therapist and the sophistication of the technology and equipment used vary enormously.

It may be disturbing and outright frightening to read about the possible complications. Nevertheless, I urge you to read and consider this information. The most experienced surgeons and the most expert radiation therapists produce the best outcomes with the lowest rates of complications. The most thoughtful and well-informed patients, in my opinion, also have the best outcomes with the lowest rates of complications. While physicians discuss and debate patient-selection criteria, you and your family should also discuss and consider carefully your treatment and physician-selection criteria. It is my hope and intention to give you the tools to do so in the chapters that follow.

8

Prostate Surgery

RADICAL PROSTATECTOMY

Radical prostatectomy is a surgical procedure in which the prostate gland, seminal vesicles, and closely associated tissue that surrounds the prostate gland are removed. Unlike a simple prostatectomy, where only a portion of the prostate and surrounding tissues are removed, the radical prostatectomy is a more extensive operation designed to remove the cancer, and any tissues into which the cancer could have spread. The word "radical" should not be a cause for alarm— it simply means complete removal of these tissues and should not be associated with the kind of disfiguring procedures women with breast cancer have to undergo with the traditional radical mastectomy.

The radical prostatectomy has historically been the treatment option most commonly chosen by patients with localized prostate cancer. This includes all stage A and B disease and certain patients with stage C disease. However, because the operation resulted in impotence in almost all the patients who underwent it, radical prostatectomies lost a great deal of popularity among both patients and surgeons in the late 1970s and 1980s.

NERVE-SPARING PROCEDURES

All that has changed due to the work of Dr. Patrick Walsh of the Johns Hopkins Hospital in Baltimore. The story underscores the importance of both high-tech discoveries and basic understanding of anatomy in leading to improved medical outcomes.

While studying in Europe, Dr. Walsh wanted to understand more fully why the majority (nearly 98 percent) of men were rendered impotent following radical prostatectomy. Of equal importance was understanding the reason why the other 2 percent were able to maintain their potency. Walsh teamed up with Dr. Donker of the Netherlands, who was performing detailed anatomic studies of the prostate gland. What emerged when the two investigators shared their information was the discovery of the more exact positions and functions of the nerves and blood vessels responsible for both getting and maintaining an erection. They discovered that during the routine surgery of removing the prostate gland, these crucial nerves and blood vessels were usually cut, rendering patients impotent. In a series of detailed surgical studies, several modifications in performing a radical prostatectomy were developed. These changes made it possible to identify and protect ("spare") these nerves and blood vessels while removing the cancerous prostate gland.

This modified procedure is now known as "nerve-sparing radical prostatectomy," "potency-sparing radical prostatectomy," or "anatomic radical prostatectomy." Since the nerves and blood vessels that supply the penis and govern erection are present on both sides of the prostate gland, the surgeon has the opportunity to spare either one side or both sides. Thus, both unilateral (one side) and bilateral (both sides) nerve-sparing operations may be discussed as options. A unilateral operation has a much lower likelihood of preserving potency.

The ability of the nerve-sparing operation to eradicate the cancer and reduce the incidence of impotence associated with the treatment has been widely acclaimed as a major breakthrough for prostate cancer patients. Through Dr. Walsh's efforts, numbers of surgeons have seen the operation or trained with him to become expert in performing the procedure. Medical articles, documentaries, and training films that outline every detail of the operation have led to the training of competent surgeons who are able to perform the procedure. But while much praise has been rightly given to Dr. Walsh and his colleagues, some prominent physicians in the field do not share Dr. Walsh's enthusiasm for the surgery.

The questions raised are: First, is the new nerve-sparing operation truly effective in controlling and eradicating the prostate cancer, or is the surgery leaving behind residual prostate cancer cells which may eventually kill the patient? Secondly, do all surgeons performing the operation achieve the same low complication rate as Dr. Walsh? As you will see, reports of the frequency of impotence as a complication vary greatly.

Patients may get conflicting information about the risk of impotency when trying to choose between radiation therapy and surgery. If the patient is less than fifty-five and has a smaller, organ-confined cancer in one lobe of the prostate gland, a bilateral nerve-sparing procedure can be performed and the likelihood of maintaining potency is quite good. A sixty-five-year-old patient with a larger cancer involving more than one lobe cannot have a bilateral nerve-sparing procedure. Here, the likelihood of maintaining potency drops dramatically. The media have tended to highlight the best possible outcomes, and these may not be realistic for all men undergoing the operation.

Judging the adequacy of the operation as a definitive cure for localized cancer is also difficult. There are surgeons who feel that the nerve-sparing approach is inadequate to maximize eradication of the cancer. These surgeons refer to cases when the gland is removed and found to contain cancer cells on the outside of the prostate gland—a so-called "dirty" or positive margin. This can certainly happen with a conventional radical prostatectomy as well, but the risk may be lower.

The major questions that still need to be answered relating to the nerve-sparing procedure include:

1.   Who is the best candidate for the operation? Clearly, the results in terms of cancer control and maintenance of potency will be much greater in a patient forty to sixty years old who has a very small tumor and who is still very much sexually active.

2.   What is the incidence of positive margins with nerve-sparing procedures compared to nonnerve-sparing procedures? This information is somewhat difficult to obtain because of disagreements about the definition of a positive margin.

3.   What are the rates of potency following a nerve-sparing procedure? Are the criteria used to define potency by one group of surgical investigators acceptable to others? Are there differing opinions regarding potency as assessed by the surgeon, the spouse, or the patient himself?

Potency is not an all-or-nothing issue. The patient may report a reduced ability to achieve and maintain an erection that the physician decides is unimportant but the spouse may consider quite significant! Very different outcomes can be claimed, and unless you are able to analyze how the information was collected and what criteria were used, it is difficult to know what it all means. Because of the ambiguities in arriving at answers to these questions, surgeons who do not favor the nerve-sparing operation will counsel their patients to undergo the traditional radical prostatectomy and deal with the consequences of impotence either postoperatively, when a variety of treatment choices can be discussed, or at the time of the prostatectomy (by using medicines or implanting a penile prosthesis). It is important to realize that nearly all men can regain their potency with various medicines or devices if they are rendered impotent from the surgery.

The issue is a complex one, and I would be misleading you if I simplified the controversy or the questions. Nonetheless, a nerve-sparing procedure is an option to be considered for younger, sexually active men with a small focal cancer, when it is performed by an experienced surgeon with a good track record.

WHAT TO EXPECT
IF YOU CHOOSE SURGERY

It is very important for the patient to understand what will happen when the operation takes place and what the postoperative recovery will be like. Understanding the complications involved is also essential for deciding for or against surgery, or which type of prostatectomy to choose.

Physicians will usually recommend that a patient scheduled for a radical prostatectomy "autodonate" blood prior to the operation. Blood loss can occur during any operative procedure, and replacement through blood bank donors always involves some level of risk. Procedures have been developed in which patients donate between two and three units of their own blood in the two to three weeks prior to the operation. This blood is reserved for use during your operation if needed. By having your own blood available for transfusion, the likelihood of requiring blood components from random donors is minimized. Your body, too, will have a chance to recover from the blood donations since a relatively small amount is taken. You should be aware that your donated blood will expire and not be usable if the operation is canceled or postponed.

On occasion, patients may receive erythropoietin, a new biotechnology product. It is a hormone that stimulates the production of red blood cells to build up the red-blood count prior to the surgery, and it may allow more blood to be donated in the period before the surgery is performed. It may also be given postsurgery as well to help the body make up any blood loss. You will have to ask your physician about receiving this hormone and its expense.

Routine preoperative testing is generally straightforward if you are considered to have no major risk factors for the surgical procedure. An electrocardiogram, chest X-ray, and routine blood and urine studies generally round out the preoperative evaluation, along with a visit with the anesthesiologist. Other specialists, such as a cardiologist, may also be consulted, depending on your age and general health. These are in addition to all the diagnostic studies performed as part of the prostate cancer evaluation.

There are two approaches to performing a radical prostatectomy: a perineal prostatectomy, in which the incision is made in the space between the scrotum and the anus (the perineum), and a retropubic prostatectomy, in which the incision is made in the lower abdomen. Some surgeons prefer the perineal approach, but it has a major disadvantage, in my view, because it does not allow sampling of the lymph nodes as part of the same operative procedure. If a perineal approach is selected, then the lymph nodes should be biopsied laporoscopically by an experienced physician as part of the diagnostic and staging procedures, or through a separate retropubic operation.

As noted in Chapter 3, most surgeons perform a lymph-node dissection as part of the retropubic radical prostatectomy. You and your physician should have an agreement ahead of time concerning what type of surgery will take place once the lymph-node status is known. In the past, most surgeons sent a lymph-node tissue sample to the pathology department for an immediate "frozen section" analysis. If the analysis showed that the lymph nodes contained no cancer, the radical prostatectomy then took place. If the frozen sections showed that the lymph nodes contained cancer, the remainder of the operation was then canceled. Additional treatment options were discussed at a later date.

The cancers that are being detected and treated today appear to be "earlier" cancers. Many surgeons continue to perform the lymph-node dissection, but they may not necessarily wait for the frozen section results, especially when the nodal tissue appears normal to the surgeon. Only when something is suspicious will the frozen section results be required before the operation proceeds. This makes reasonable sense given our improved ability to predict the likelihood of positive nodes when the Gleason grade of the biopsy, the clinical stage of the patient, and the PSA are all factored into the decision. Some surgeons are no longer performing the lymph-node dissection in selected patients considered to have an extremely low risk of harboring lymph node metastases.

A prior understanding must be established between surgeon and patient about what will be done if the lymph nodes are found to contain cancer. There are instances when the surgeon will opt to proceed with the radical prostatectomy, even when there is known metastatic disease in the nodes. While most surgeons do not agree with performing a radical prostatectomy when metastatic disease is found, the possibility must be discussed prior to the operation, You need to understand fully the reasons why the radical prostatectomy will or will not be performed.

There are some case reports (not proven by rigorous scientific study) to support performing a radical prostatectomy in the patient with minimal involvement of only one lymph node. These reports suggest that patients with limited, microscopic involvement may have the same favorable outcome as patients undergoing the operation who did not have lymph node involvement. Other reports suggest that the immediate institution of hormonal therapy in the node-positive patient who has undergone a radical prostatectomy may result in an excellent outcome. Be aware, however, that these results are not universally accepted or acknowledged as reliable.

If you decide on a nerve-sparing procedure, you should have a discussion with your surgeon in advance concerning how vigorously the surgeon will try to spare the nerves and vessels needed for an erection. Since our preoperative evaluations are usually not precise, the findings during the actual operation may dictate a different operation than that agreed upon preoperatively. If suspicious areas are found during the operation, if it is not a small, organ-confined tumor, then the neurovascular areas may have to be sacrificed, reducing the likelihood of preserving potency, but maximizing your chance of eliminating the cancer.

In the best of all worlds, a patient who has a radical prostatectomy can expect to be in the hospital for three to seven days. This length is an average and applies to hospitalizations in which there are no complications. If there are any complications you may expect to stay longer.

COMPLICATIONS OF PROSTATE SURGERY

Most of the complications associated with prostate surgery are long-term or late complications—those that persist for some time after discharge from the hospital. Complications that occur during hospitalization can be related to the surgery itself, or to complications of anesthesia, and are not specific to prostate cancer surgery. Those related to the surgery include blood loss that requires blood transfusions. With any surgery, infections at the site of the incision can occur and may require drainage of infected fluids.

One of the most significant complications of surgery in the postoperative period is the development of blood clots. Because most patients who have prostate cancer surgery are active men in otherwise excellent health, when such a patient is suddenly kept immobilized in bed during the postoperative hospitalization the blood flow through the body can be altered. The circulating blood can become more static, and more prone to clotting or congealing. Prostate surgery, along with other major abdominal procedures, appears to encourage the formation of clots.

Clotting is most likely to happen in the legs. The earliest symptom of a blood clot is a tender, swollen leg, happening within days to a week following the operation. The condition, called thrombophlebitis, is treated with bedrest and often with the administration of blood-thinning agents. A blood clot that is dislodged and carried through the bloodstream until it blocks an artery is called an embolus, and the event is called embolism. Pulmonary embolism, in which blood clots travel to the lung to block the pulmonary artery, is an emergency condition. The common symptoms of a pulmonary embolus are acute shortness of breath and chest pain. A pulmonary embolus can cause death if the clot is large, or if heart and lung function are weakened.

Fortunately, the diagnosis of a pulmonary embolus is relatively straightforward and can be treated with blood-thinning agents. Blood clots can significantly prolong the hospitalization period. Although hospital personnel are constantly checking for blood-clot symptoms in a patient after surgery, the patient can often help to decrease the risk of having clots form. One simple maneuver is to continually flex your legs while lying in bed after surgery. Wearing special stockings can also diminish risk. Low doses of blood-thinning agents (heparin) are often used as a preventive measure. However, on occasion fluid collections may occur in the abdomen, and require drainage.

In a prostatectomy, there is always a possibility that structures near the prostate gland may be damaged during the surgery. Although rare, these complications can occur and can include damage to the rectum, ureter, or the nerves of the pelvis. Any surgical injury may increase the hospitalization time, and, on occasion, require additional surgery to repair the damage. Finally, although rare, death from surgery occurs in 0.1 percent to 0.8 percent of patients.

Table 4. Complications of Radical Prostatectomy

Short-term complications

Blood Loss
Incontinence (short term)
Blood clotting leading to phlebitis or embolism
Injuries to surrounding structures
Wound infections and fluid collections
Heart- or lung-function complications resulting
       from anesthesia or surgery

Late-term complications

Impotence
Incontinence

Evaluate the Surgeon, Not Just the Surgery

There are statistics available for the incidence of these different complications and these incidence rates can be helpful in deciding for or against prostate surgery, or any of the other available treatments. However, it is crucial to remember that surgery is a skill, and the really important statistics are those for the surgeon rather than the surgery. You must ask the surgeon, before he or she becomes your surgeon, these four essential questions (you will doubtlessly think of others):

1. How many of these procedures have you performed?
2. What is the average length of hospitalization?
3. What is the incidence of complications in your patients?
4. Specifically, what is your patients' incidence of incontinence? Impotence?

In some regions of the country, hospitals report their complication rates for different surgical procedures annually, and this information is published or made available in one form or another. You may be able to access this information with the help of a community librarian.

Incontinence

Incontinence is a dreaded complication and is often the most influential consideration when a patient selects one type of treatment over another. Incontinence is often misunderstood by both physician and patient. There have been several surveys where the patient was asked questions regarding the presence and severity of incontinence following radical prostatectomy. The physician performing the operation was also asked to make a similar assessment. To no one's surprise there was a great disparity in the reported results. In one survey, patients reported a 30 percent incidence of incontinence, yet their physicians only reported an incidence of 1 percent to 2 percent.

Such a communication breakdown underscores the importance of straight talk and proper explanation between health-care provider and patient. While a physician may not think a little dampness is a major calamity, the uninformed patient may consider this a totally unexpected outcome that has changed his lifestyle. This risk and the frequency of this complication needs to be fully understood by the patient prior to the operation.

Remember the anatomy of the prostate gland as described in Chapter 2 and the fact that it surrounds the urethra, which carries urine from the bladder. Under normal circumstances, passage of urine through the urethra is under the control of sphincters or valves, which open and close at precise times corresponding to the urge to urinate. The portion of the urethra that passes through the prostate gland must be reconnected following removal of the prostate gland. It is a delicate connection and includes, among other things, the reconnection of tissues that affect a sphincter that controls urine flow. Any surgery in this area is likely to cause swelling and some temporary dysfunction which may result in involuntary loss of urine, or incontinence. In addition, it takes several months, and sometimes as much as a year, to recondition the muscular sphincter that controls the flow of urine.

As a result, it is very common for patients to complain of "stress" incontinence following the operation. Stress in this case means force exerted on the abdominal muscles, as in coughing or sneezing, or pushing at the time of a bowel movement (straining at stool). Under these abdominal stresses, the sphincter is not strong enough to hold the urine in, and some drips out. Fortunately, this condition is short-lived, lasting from weeks to several months. Although common, postprostatectomy incontinence should still be evaluated by your physician, since urinary tract infection or urinary retention, rather than the surgery, could be the underlying cause.

Depending on the degree and duration of the incontinence, it can be managed by wearing absorbent pads, the use of nonpainful clamps on the penis, wearing a device called a condom catheter, or by an indwelling catheter for a short time postdischarge. Recovery of sphincter tone can be helped with a program of Keegel exercises, which help strengthen the sphincter. But it takes time, and my best advice is to be patient.

About 5 percent to 10 percent of patients will have persistent incontinence, and these need a detailed diagnostic evaluation to determine the cause and most appropriate treatment. Anticholinergic drugs, behavior modification, biofeedback, and electrical stimulation can all be useful treatments for incontinence resulting from involuntary contractions of the detrusor muscle of the bladder, which is responsible for pushing the urine out of the bladder.

More definitive treatments are necessary if the sphincter was damaged in the surgery, the incontinence is more severe, and the patient is constantly wet because of urinary leakage. Here, more active intervention by urologists skilled in reconstructive techniques may be required. One promising treatment that is still considered investigational involves the injections of "biocompatible" substances such as collagen or teflon into the area surrounding the urethra. These "bulking agents" serve to increase the urethra's resistance to urine flow. Another effective option is the surgical implantation of an artificial urethral sphincter that the patient controls to urinate as necessary.

If you do have persistent or severe incontinence, it is important for you to seek treatment. You ultimately are the one who must decide if the incontinence you are experiencing is causing you distress and diminishing your quality of life. If it is limiting your daily activities and you feel your physician minimizes your concern and is not offering solutions, then you are justified in seeking another opinion.

Impotence

Since millions of men in the United States are estimated to suffer from impotence, a large portion of those who develop prostate cancer may well suffer from some degree of sexual dysfunction at the time of diagnosis. Since nearly every treatment for prostate cancer is likely to diminish sexual functioning, and many patients with partial erectile dysfunction have not been fully evaluated before treatment, comparison of treatment results and complication rates is very problematic.

Also, there is no standardized method of questioning patients and their partners about sexual functioning. The way a surgeon evaluates sexual functioning after a nerve-sparing radical prostatectomy may be different from the assessment of another health-care provider or, more importantly, the patient himself. Studies are now being made in which treatment "success" is independently evaluated by the medical team (or more commonly, the individual physician doing the research) and the patient. The results of such studies are revealing.

In one recent evaluation, in which surgeons and the patients were asked about the adequacy of sexual functioning following surgery, the physician response to the question was 50 percent to 70 percent for the series of surgeries studied. When the same question was asked of the patient and sexual partner, a much lower 30 percent reported a satisfactory outcome.

In a series of nearly a thousand patients who received Medicare benefits and had undergone radical prostatectomy (either traditional or nerve-sparing), nearly 90 percent responded that they had been able to have an erection adequate for sexual intercourse prior to their surgery. Following surgery, nearly 60 percent of those in the study stated that they had been unable to attain either a partial or full erection necessary for intercourse since the surgery. Only 11 percent of patients stated that they were able to achieve an erection of sufficient hardness to have intercourse. However, it is important to consider that these patients may have been somewhat older than average, and not all would have received a nerve-sparing radical prostatectomy.

THE UNEXPECTED

Sometimes healthy patients in the care of experienced surgeons and hospital staff can develop unforeseeable complications. Daniel Husik, a patient discussed in more detail in Chapter 11, experienced a massive amount of bleeding during surgery and in the immediate postoperative period in the recovery room. He required nearly eleven units of blood (a unit is equal to about one pint of blood) and massive amounts of other fluids to maintain his blood pressure and replace the blood that was lost during the operation. His pre- and postoperative blood studies did not demonstrate any blood-function abnormalities, and it remains unclear why he lost so much blood during the operation.

Douglas Fiedler, a patient who many experts would have considered for watchful waiting, experienced a severe postoperative infection of the intestinal tract which prolonged his hospitalization by a week plus an additional three to four weeks of convalescence at home. The primary problem was a delay in determining the type of bacteria present, which were causing severe diarrhea. When the bacteria was identified and treated with the appropriate antibiotics, there was a rapid response.

The reason for paying so much attention to the topic of complications and to the experiences of these latter two patients is to emphasize the stark fact that complications do occur in the finest of hospitals—both community-based and university. You and your family should factor the possibility of such complications into your decision-making and planning. The ideal hospitalization in which the patient is admitted, operated upon, and discharged without any short-term complications does happen, but cannot be counted on in every case.

9

RADIATION THERAPY

The second major modality for treating localized prostate cancer is with radiation therapy, also called radiotherapy. This chapter will tell you what you need to know about radiation therapy to evaluate this treatment option.

The use of radiation damages cancer cells, rendering them unable to undergo continued cell growth and division. In contrast to normal cells, cancer cells are unlikely to be able to repair the damage that results from the radiation treatments, and thus the cancer cells eventually die.

There are two main ways of delivering radiation treatments to the gland. The first and more common is called external-beam radiotherapy. The second is known as radioactive prostate seed implantation, interstitial radiotherapy, or brachytherapy. In the first the source of the radiation is external; in the second, the radioactive material is implanted in the prostate gland itself. (If you're interested, the Greek prefix *brachy* is pronounced "brak-ee" and means "short." The sense is that in brachytherapy the radiation is located a short distance from the target tissue.)

EXTERNAL-BEAM RADIOTHERAPY

In the most commonly applied situation, a very sophisticated machine called a linear accelerator is used to produce a focused, high-energy X-ray beam. The patient is placed into the machine, and utilizing precise physics, computer applications, and mechanical-engineering principles, a carefully calculated portion of the radiation (the radiation dose) is aimed at the cancerous tissues in the prostate gland. To minimize the damage to normal tissue, treatments are given over a period of several weeks with gradual increases in the radiation dose (sometimes called fractionation of dose). Such a practice allows the normal tissue to repair itself in between the treatments.

Complications, discussed below, relate mainly to damage done to vital tissue in the rectum, resulting in irritation, blood loss, and diarrhea of varying degrees of severity. There have been several technical advances in radiation therapy for localized prostate cancer that should help to limit the frequency and severity of these complications. New techniques now better define the specific "volume" of cancer to be irradiated and diminish the exposure of surrounding normal tissues. Computer simulations of the exact anatomic position of the individual prostate gland allow more precise focusing of the beam to "hit" the target areas. This increased precision can allow the ever-increasing doses of radiation to be more precisely targeted to the cancerous tissue, thereby improving the possibility of cancer elimination. Such techniques are called *three-dimensional conformal* radiation. The preliminary results suggest excellent cancer control with fewer side effects, but no long-term results are available.

BRACHYTHERAPY

The second major type of radiation treatment for prostate cancer is called interstitial radiotherapy, or brachytherapy. Instead of having an external beam of radiation generated by a machine, individual seeds or pellets of radioactive material are surgically implanted (placed into) the prostate gland itself. Once commonly done, brachytherapy fell out of favor as a treatment because of early technical difficulties with how the pellets were delivered to the tissue. Improved techniques that allow a more precise delivery of the pellets to the cancerous areas has led to new interest in this treatment approach. The long-term results of using these newer radioactive sources and more sophisticated placement of the seeds are not available, since these technical advances are so recent.

The sources of radiation originally used were radioactive iodine or gold. Today, different sources of radiation are used and include palladium and others. Often brachytherapy patients also receive external-beam radiation as a supplement. By combining these two types of radiation treatments, there is a greater assurance that the proper dose of radiation has been given to the cancer.

From a patient's perspective, there are less severe side effects associated with brachytherapy, and in certain circumstances a larger number of patients are able to maintain their potency compared to either external-beam radiation therapy or surgery. At a recent conference sponsored by the American Cancer Society that focused on understanding patient preferences, many patients expressed great acceptance of interstitial brachytherapy despite the fact that long-term follow-up results are not yet available.

The older form of brachytherapy, in which the radioactive seeds were implanted into the prostate "freehand," was associated with inferior results in terms of localized cancer control in patients with palpable prostate cancers. The long-term outcomes for these early patients were recently analyzed by two of my colleagues, Dr. Anthony D'Amico and Dr. Norman Coleman, both radiation oncologists practicing at Harvard Medical School. When compared to external-beam radiation therapy, the use of implanted seeds did not eradicate or control the cancer in the prostate gland area in 17 percent to 52 percent of patients with stage B disease. In contrast, comparable local failure rates in traditionally treated external-beam radiation patients ranged from 4 percent to 13 percent. When patients with stage C disease were studied, the local failure rates were nearly two to three times greater in the interstitial implanted patients than the external-beam patients.

Again, the technique used in the earlier form of brachytherapy is quite inferior to that used today. The seeds were placed into the prostate gland without a scientific way of measuring if the tumor was receiving the correct dose. Moreover, if the radioactive seeds were positioned too close to the capsule or too close to the urethra, damage was likely to occur to either the rectum or the urethra. These complications could be quite debilitating, resulting in the need for a colostomy (diversion of the bowel and fecal contents to an outside bag) or the surgical reestablishment of urinary flow.

Recent studies have lead to a reevaluation of brachytherapy. Several major factors have caused such a resurgence in interest, and will be of great importance when you are trying to evaluate whether you are a candidate for this procedure.

The first relates to better visualization of the individual prostate gland at the time of seed implantation. With the use of CT scanning of the prostate gland, and improved TRUS techniques, the prostate can be nicely visualized. Specifically, the location of the urethra and the prostate capsule can be understood. Thus, the radioactive seeds can be more accurately positioned to avoid dangerously high doses of radiation to the surrounding normal structures, the major cause of complications with the older technique. Despite accurate initial placement, however, the seeds are not "anchored" in the prostate and can migrate to a different part of the gland with the result being that some areas of the prostate may receive suboptimal radiation dosage.

Second, there is a better understanding of which patients are most likely to benefit from the procedure. Past studies have not relied upon the use of PSA in determining which patients should be treated. Now by using sophisticated probability curves calculated from a large body of long-term data, we can help predict better than before which patients are likely to have organ-confined versus nonorgan-confined (and more extensive) disease. Thus, physicians can "select" patients who are more likely to get a good result in terms of cancer control and a lower incidence of complications, including impotency.

Several patient characteristics emerge for the "ideal" brachytherapy patient. He is generally sexually active, has a nonpalpable cancer usually picked up by PSA-based screening, has a Gleason score of between 2 to 4, and had a PSA value of under 10 ng/ml. The likelihood of this patient having a cancer which is confined to the prostate gland, without either capsular penetration or "positive margins," is about 75 percent. By selecting this type of patient, the radiotherapist, radiologist, and surgeon, working as a team, can hope to maximize the delivery of the appropriate dose to the gland to maintain potency and eradicate the cancer. We cannot, however, state that these goals have been achieved. The follow-up of these patient groups has been too short to provide definitive data.

After publication of my April 1994 article, "The Dilemmas of Prostate Cancer," in *Scientific American*, I received a letter from a reader taking me to task for not giving more attention to brachytherapy in my article. Describing his own experiences with prostate cancer he wrote:

As a 68-year-old sexually active male, the diagnosis of prostate cancer was emotionally devastating. I had no symptoms but a routine physical followed by a PSA blood test and then a biopsy resulted in a phone call. "I'm sorry," said the urologist, "but you seem to be one of the unlucky ones." He told me to bank some blood, get CAT and bone scans, and said he would reserve a hospital space five weeks hence. I was too numb to resent his arrogance.

I consulted four other MDs. Their only options for my stage B, moderately aggressive cancer were surgery or external-beam radiation. One of the surgeons urged me to "go for the cure." A radiation therapist commented that it was dark and slippery down there and surgery might miss some of the cancer.

Fortunately, I also consulted a urologist at the _____ Hospital. After listening to my concerns about potency and continence, he suggested brachytherapy, the implantation of radioactive seeds directly in the prostate. I entered the hospital in the morning and 75 Iodine 125 pellets were inserted under general anesthetic. Late that same afternoon I returned home under my own power. After a couple of days I was back to normal. That was two years ago. Today my PSA is low and my quality of life high.

The author of this letter makes some important points (including the insensitivity all too often shown by physicians), and he has enjoyed an excellent short-term outcome. Once again, though, the long-term efficacy of the new techniques are not yet known. With the older, less reliable method of implanting the radioactive pellets, the cumulative experience has not been entirely positive. Long-term results have failed to show improvements in survival or local control compared to more conventional modalities. This does not mean that the procedure of interstitial implantation of radioactive seeds should not be recommended. It may be an excellent treatment in appropriate circumstances, as illustrated by the above letter.

The short-term data are encouraging. Nearly 70 to 80 percent of patients with early prostate cancer (stage A and some stage B) may be free of cancer, with a normal PSA test three years after the procedure. However, the selection of "favorable disease" needs to be emphasized here, along with the small number of patients for whom these excellent results are obtainable. The ability to maintain potency is also reported to be high in this group of patients, with some figures being as high as 70 percent. The bad news in these early results, however, is the occurrence of bowel and urinary complications. Despite selecting younger, healthier patients who were likely to achieve a good result, there have been significant instances when patients have suffered radiation damage to either the urethra or the rectum, necessitating additional corrective surgeries.

My advice at this juncture is to be aware of interstitial therapy as yet another alternative for the treatment of localized prostate cancer. Here again, the selection of a team that does this treatment on a regular basis, and has expertise in visualizing and targeting the prostate gland during the implantation procedure is going to be a critical component in increasing the odds of having a favorable result. It is also important to see the published (or documented) outcomes of the hospital facility and the physician before selecting an individual health-care provider.

All too often, early results of a new procedure will be accompanied with a higher degree of complications. A "learning curve" is established, and later results generated by the dedicated team can in fact be better (hopefully so) than the early results. A health-care facility just starting to perform the new procedure after a second wave of more favorable outcomes have been published may quote these improved statistics to you. While this may be helpful for you to get a better picture of what is going on, these more favorable figures may have no applicability to the actual institution where you are considering being treated! The implantation of these radioactive pellets is technically challenging, and not to be undertaken lightly by the inexperienced operator. Also, we have no data to date on the results of follow-up biopsies following brachytherapy. Until such data is available, brachytherapy is best considered a promising but not confirmed treatment for localized prostate cancer.

WHO SHOULD CHOOSE RADIOTHERAPY?

Patients who have a prostate cancer which can be appropriately treated with either radiation or surgery will have to weigh all the evidence of both efficacy and side effects in making a decision. The patient with risk factors for developing complications associated with one treatment should select the program which is least likely to result in treatment-related harm.

Because of the inherent risks of surgery, older men and men with other serious medical conditions usually receive radiation therapy. As a result, the total population of patients with localized prostate cancer who are treated with radiation therapy are more likely to be in poorer health than the total population of patients who opt for surgery. When statistics are compared, patients who are treated with radiation therapy have a lower five-year survival rate than surgically treated patients.

However, these sicker patients who received radiation therapy may not routinely die of prostate cancer; they may die from another condition. When these general mortality statistics are misinterpreted, as is often done, they are viewed as a demonstration of the superiority of surgery over radiation treatments, even though the differences were due to the fact that a generally sicker group of patients was selected for radiation treatment. When death rates due specifically to prostate cancer in both surgically treated and radiation-treated populations are compared, the differences are much less compared to survival rates which don't distinguish the specific reasons for death.

WHAT TO EXPECT IF YOU CHOOSE RADIATION THERAPY

If you choose external-beam radiation therapy, you will normally have a CT scan of the prostate and perhaps other tests to gather the data needed for the simulation. This is a computerized three-dimensional representation of your body that is done by a radiation physicist. It is used to study your individual anatomy, to select the treatment fields (the abnormal tissues the radiation will target), and to guide the construction of the shielding blocks that will be used to protect your normal tissues from radiation damage.

For each treatment you will be placed on the table of the linear accelerator in precisely the same position with the shielding blocks in place. Several other steps are often taken to ensure that your body position is exactly the same for each treatment. For example, tattoos may be used to help guide beam placement. It is now common to try to have the patient's bladder be the same every day to avoid variations in the prostate gland's position in relation to the balloonlike bladder. So, you may be asked to come for treatment with a full bladder, or given other instructions to help keep bladder distension as uniform as possible.

Treatments generally take about 15 minutes and are usually performed by a technician. You will see your radiation therapist weekly during the course of treatment under most circumstances. The treatments are usually done five days a week for about seven weeks, but do not be surprised if your schedule is different for one reason or another. Before and during treatment your blood-cell counts will be taken to watch for drops in counts that may require a break in treatments. A "sunburn-like" feeling around the anus or the buttocks is not unusual as a result of treatment. An antinausea medicine may be prescribed to treat nausea resulting from the radiation treatments.

COMPLICATIONS OF RADIATION THERAPY

Because of the complications and risks of surgery, radiation therapy is usually the preferred option for a patient with other medical conditions. Radiation therapy, however, also has risks and complications, shown in Table 5. Impotence and incontinence can result from this treatment, as from surgery, because of damage to the same tissues. However, there is a greater likelihood of regaining potency after the end of the treatments.

Proctitis, or inflammation of the lower rectal area, is one of the most common complications of external-beam radiation therapy, and can be mild or severe. Because of the close proximity of the prostate gland to the rectum, it is often technically difficult to "spare" the normal tissue (the rectal lining) from the "target" tissue (the prostate gland) containing the cancer. Thus the normal tissues suffer some radiation damage. If this occurs in the bladder, patients will complain of bladder irritation or pain upon urination. When it occurs in the lower rectum, diarrhea results. A break in the treatment usually allows healing, and shortly thereafter, treatments can resume.

There is a relative lack of serious complications associated with brachytherapy, a major reason for its growing popularity, along with the ease and convenience of the treatment. Radiation damage to the rectum or bladder does occur, as discussed above. Both with conformal external-beam radiation and brachytherapy, the improved techniques now available should reduce the severity and frequency of these complications. Because these technical improvements are relatively new, you must be very careful to find out whether the technology and expertise needed are in fact available at the institution where you wish to be treated.

Table 5. Complications of Radiation Therapy

Proctitis (inflammation of the rectum, which may
      result in bloody diarrhea)
Cystitis (inflammation of the bladder, sometimes
      leading to bloody or painful urination)
Impotence
Swelling around the penis and scrotum
Long-term chronic diarrhea
Difficulty in urination
Urinary incontinence
Bowel blockage or obstruction

TREATMENT FAILURES

In the controversies over the superiority of surgery versus radiation as definitive treatments, surgeons often point to the fact that studies have shown a significant number of positive biopsies within the year and a half after definitive radiation treatments. However, it is not certain whether the cancerous cells found in the postradiation biopsies are actually viable—capable of dividing to grow more cancer. "Treatment failures"—disease recurrence one, five, ten, or even fifteen years after treatment—can occur with either surgery or radiation. The recurrence can be caused by residual disease that was missed, or by metastatic disease that was undetectable at the time of treatment.

If there is a positive margin or other evidence of definite residual disease following surgery, the treatment options for that patient include radiation treatments. However, conventional surgery is difficult in the radiation-treated patient who has residual disease in the prostate or neighboring tissues detected on later testing. This is because radiation treatments leave behind a mass of unrecognizable scar tissue that is difficult to "resect"—to remove surgically—without a great deal of bleeding and potential damage to vital tissues. For this reason, radiation-treated patients with residual cancer in the gland are potential candidates for hormonal therapy or for cryosurgery, discussed in the following chapter. However, some surgeons are performing radical prostatectomies on increasing number of patients previously treated with 3D conformal radiation therapy but in whom the cancer has recurred in the prostate area. It seems that the amount of scarring and scar tissue formation may be less in patients treated with 3D conformal radiation as compared to conventional radiation, thus making the surgery easier.

THE UNEXPECTED

At various points, I discuss patients who received radiation therapy following neoadjuvant hormonal therapy (described in the following chapter) or after surgery because of a positive margin. These patients, Wilson Orr and Daniel Husik, experienced few or tolerable side effects and to date are doing very well. Stephen Fisher, discussed in Chapter 12, "Sexual Issues," opted for radiation therapy because of the greater likelihood that he would regain his potency after treatment. He also achieved excellent results in terms of tolerable side effects and short-term efficacy. As he hoped, he was able to become sexually active again following treatment. The experiences of Samuel Taggert unfortunately illustrate a poor outcome occurring in a sicker patient who would not have been considered for surgery.

Mr. Taggert learned he had prostate cancer after participating in a public screening program during Prostate Cancer Awareness Week in 1990. An elevated PSA value prompted a DRE, which was abnormal. He was diagnosed with locally confined Stage B1, Gleason 3 + 3 carcinoma. Since he was only sixty-two years old at the time of this diagnosis, Mr. Taggert might have been considered for either surgery or radiation with a good expectation of cure. However, his evaluation revealed considerable impairment of lung function, and a detailed history revealed that the patient had moderately severe emphysema, making any surgery a risky undertaking. His urologist and a pulmonary (lung) consultant felt that the treatment of choice was external-beam radiation therapy rather than a radical prostatectomy. Both felt that Mr. Taggert's poor lung function put him at greater risk of disability or death than his cancer. For this reason, a policy of nonintervention (watchful waiting or observation) was also discussed, but this option was rejected by both the patient and his spouse. After a lengthy discussion, the decision to select radiation treatments was made.

Because he and his family wanted to stay in the Florida for the winter and spring months, Mr. Taggert opted to have treatment given at a local hospital near his Florida home. The treatments occurred over a period of seven weeks and were complicated by several unplanned "treatment breaks" when treatments were temporarily suspended (usually for a period of seven to ten days) to allow some healing of damaged tissue that was within the irradiated field (the area targeted by the beam). In Mr. Taggert's case, the breaks were required for proctitis, causing diarrhea and irritation to his rectum. The treatment breaks are intended to give the tissues time to heal. In about 3 percent of cases, the diarrhea does not resolve, and patients are then faced with having surgery to repair the bowel damage, or learning to live with a fairly intolerable situation. Such was the case with Mr. Taggert.

Treatment was eventually completed, and Mr. Taggert had a very nice response in terms of curing his cancer. His PSA fell to a normal range and his prostate gland abnormalities resolved (disappeared). About six months following completion of radiation, he began to experience fairly debilitating bloody diarrhea similar in nature to the type that required the initial treatment breaks. Treatment with cortisone-type enemas failed to provide any long-term relief. An evaluation by a gastroenterologist confirmed the presence of the lower bowel (rectum) irritation caused by the radiation treatments.

Over the next two years, Mr. Taggert's main problems stemmed from his worsening pulmonary emphysema and his radiation proctitis with bloody diarrhea that was very difficult to control. The blood loss was so severe that he even became anemic. Because red blood cells carry important oxygen throughout the body, and because his already diseased lungs were unable to carry enough oxygen, he suffered from severe fatigue. Eventually, Mr. Taggert's lung function deteriorated so substantially that he required continuous respiratory support. He became bedridden, and died of progressive lung failure nearly three years after his initial diagnosis of prostate cancer.

Should Mr. Taggert have been treated at all? The dilemma of screening, as it applies to Mr. Taggert, is seen in Figure 10. A critic of overly aggressive intervention for early prostate cancer could argue that Mr. Taggert should have had nothing done for his prostate cancer. His underlying lung disease was so severe that it predicted a low likelihood

Figure 10

THE DILEMMA OF SCREENING

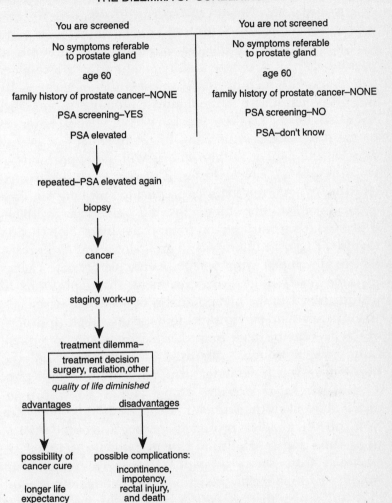

of his living another ten years. Those who argue for watchful waiting will say that his prostate cancer would not cause any substantial difficulties for ten to twelve years. Therefore, with a limited life expectancy and a slow-growing tumor, why would anyone want to actively treat this patient, given the potential side effects of treatment, which in this case were quite debilitating?

However, Mr. Taggert was a man of sixty-two, not seventy-two or eighty-two. Statistically, the older patient is more likely to die of an unrelated cause than to succumb to prostate cancer. A different story emerges for the younger patient, even though he may have coexisting medical conditions. A policy of no treatment intervention may sound rational when the decision is made, but what if medical advances in the next several years allow better treatment or even a cure for the patient's other illness? Will the opportunity to cure his prostate cancer be lost if the patient is not treated early on? What if the statistics predicting how long Mr. Taggert was going to live with emphysema were incorrect? What if he lived for six rather than three years, and the prediction that Mr. Taggert's tumor would grow slowly was also wrong, and he developed symptomatic, metastatic prostate cancer in three years? By delaying treatment, the opportunity to provide him with the highest quality of life would have been lost. There are no easy answers to these questions. Appropriate choices can be made only after patient, family, and physicians have thoroughly discussed and considered all the possibilities, which did in fact happen in Mr. Taggert's case.

Did Mr. Taggert receive proper and appropriate treatment? More likely than not, Mr. Taggert would probably not have survived a radical prostatectomy because of the severity of his lung disease. He is the type of patient who is actively excluded from series of patients who are treated with surgery. External-beam radiation was the treatment most likely to provide the best cancer control with fewer and less severe side effects.

Were the radiation treatments given using the best available technology and expertise? The answer to this question is unknown. Mr. Taggert and his wife made the decision to seek treatment at a hospital near their winter home. This hospital may well have an excellent track record with external-beam radiation, but I do not know whether the Taggerts researched this issue. It may be the case that the generally low incidence of severe long-term complications encouraged them to believe that the treatment was safe and that all radiology departments and all radiotherapists are the same.

Unfortunately, there can be substantial differences in quality, technology, and expertise, especially in demanding high-tech specialties such as radiation therapy. The type and quality of machine used to deliver the radiation doses, the techniques involved in shielding adjacent healthy tissues from the radiation beam, the planning techniques for determining the dose and the treatment intervals—all contribute to whether a patient gets a "good" result or a "less good" result.

I am in no way stating that Mr. Taggert's devastating complication of radiation proctitis was caused by inadequacies in the technical aspects of delivering radiation treatments. What I am saying is that attention to details and the genuine quality of the team providing the treatments can make an enormous difference in patient outcomes. Physicians know this and deal with it on a day-to-day basis. Referrals to competent colleagues are routine, and physicians who have higher complication rates, assuming all else is equal, are generally avoided.

The difficulty comes in when you, the patient, refer yourself to a specialist, after being seen by a local physician, and pose the question, "Doctor, where should I have my radiation therapy given?" or "Where shall I have my surgery performed?" or "Is Dr. So and So the right person to be caring for me?" These are straightforward questions, but you may not get a straightforward answer, either because the answer is not known, or because a frank answer may bring up a less-than-complimentary commentary on another physician's competence, compassion, or style.

Specialty medical societies and state medical agencies are

trying to establish standards of quality assurance and quality control for their specialities. A group of radiation oncologists has made a commendable effort to scientifically assess the quality of radiation treatments for prostate cancer over the last several decades. Studies such as this one, known as the Patterns of Care Research Effort, organized by Dr. Gerald Hanks of the Fox Chase Cancer Center in Philadelphia, have gone a long way in identifying deficiencies in radiation treatments. Attempts to correct these deficiencies and raise the overall level of competence are a constant and ongoing endeavor. Other specialties such as surgery and oncology also continue to monitor and assess the quality of treatment they provide for prostate cancer.

My general recommendation, once again, is to urge the patient to discuss specific details relating to complication rates and outcomes with the medical oncologist, surgeon, or radiologist—with whoever will be providing your care. This type of conversation can be important in helping establish rapport and mutual respect between you and your physician. A patient who develops an unexpected complication that was either not discussed or inadequately understood is very likely to become angry. In contrast, a potential or probable complication that has been extensively discussed and well understood by both the patient and his family is more likely to be thought of as an unfortunate occurrence, not a terrible mistake. I urge this type of dialogue for the benefit of patients and physicians alike.

10

Investigational and Nonstandard Therapies

With radical prostatectomy and external-beam radiation therapy, we have several decades of information as a guide to knowing what to expect—which patients are most likely to achieve the best results, what complications are to be expected, and what the long-term outcomes are likely to be for patients with different stages and grades of disease. With the newer nerve-sparing procedures and especially with brachytherapy and cryosurgery, we have more limited long-term information, but because adequate numbers of patients have received these treatments, we have some good short-term data to guide treatment selection. How are the informed patient and physician going to assess the potential good or harm offered by a therapy which is still emerging and unproven, but possibly quite beneficial? This chapter reviews some additional "nonstandard" treatment options that might offer advantages to certain patients.

NEOADJUVANT HORMONAL THERAPY

Hormonal therapy, described in Chapters 5 and 13, has long been the standard treatment for stage D metastatic cancer, cancer that cannot be cured with localized treatment such as radiation and surgery. Yet it also has potential value for stage B or C disease as an *adjuvant* therapy (an auxiliary treatment following radiation or surgery) and as a *neoadjuvant* therapy (an auxiliary treatment that precedes the definitive radiation or surgery treatment). (See Figure 11.) As an adjuvant treatment, it is sometimes used on an individual basis following a radical prostatectomy when a positive margin suggests a high likelihood of cancer recurrence.

Figure 11
ADJUVANT THERAPY

Breast

Tumor removed
lymph nodes positive

Systematic therapy
(chemotherapy or
hormonal therapy)
ADJUVANT THERAPY

Prostate

Tumor removed
lymph nodes
positive

Systematic therapy
(hormonal therapy)
ADJUVANT THERAPY

NEOADJUVANT THERAPY

Prostate

Tumor biopsied
other studies normal

Systematic therapy
(hormonal therapy)
NEOADJUVANT THERAPY

Tumor removed or
treated with
radiation after or
during hormonal
therapy

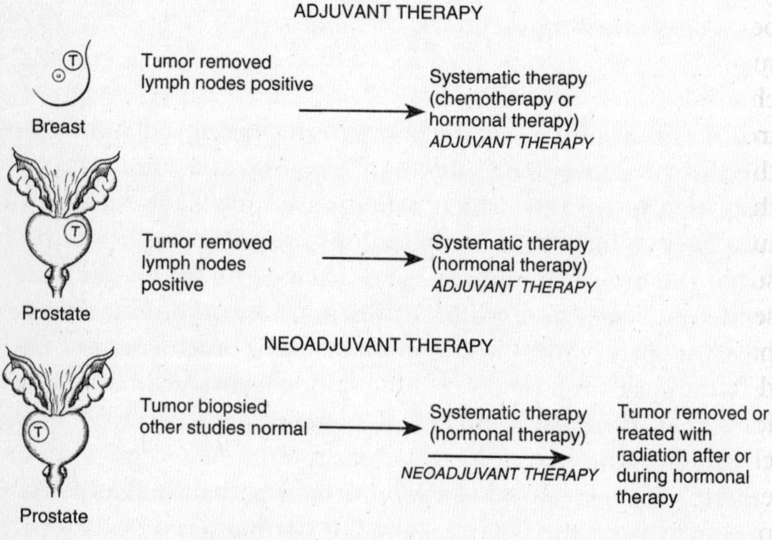

Neoadjuvant hormonal therapy is undertaken as a preliminary treatment for localized or regionally advanced prostate cancer prior to definitive treatments with either radical prostatectomy or radiation therapy. The idea is to decrease the "tumor burden"—both the size of the primary tumor and any undetected micrometastases—and thereby increase the chances of having the cancer confined to the gland at the time of surgery or radiation. When you recall the problem with clinical understaging—the fact that stage A2 and stage B and C cancers often turn out to be more advanced at the time of surgery—you can see the potential advantage to a preliminary therapy aimed at eliminating micrometastatic cancer and shrinking the primary tumor, to increase the chance that localized treatment will indeed be curative.

The use of adjuvant and neoadjuvant chemotherapy is well established for some other types of cancer. For example, adjuvant chemotherapy is given to women with breast cancer who have evidence of micrometastatic disease in the lymph nodes of the armpit. This is an "adjuvant" treatment because the primary cancer in the breast has been either surgically removed or irradiated before the systemic chemotherapy begins. In the case of bladder cancer, newer treatment programs use combination "neoadjuvant" chemotherapy prior to either radiation or surgery to "downstage" the primary cancer. In certain circumstances, the bladder tumors have been so significantly downstaged that lesser surgery has been required, even enabling patients to preserve their bladders. Patients with testicular cancer often have large metastatic deposits present in the back of the abdomen resulting from testis cancer that has traveled and lodged in the lymph nodes. In such instances, the use of chemotherapy will significantly decrease the size of the masses, enabling the surgeon to remove them. A substantial number of patients given this neoadjuvant therapy will have negative lymph nodes at the time of surgery. Here, chemotherapy has been able to "sterilize" these large masses, or has converted them to a less formidable and less aggressive type of cancer.

We do not yet have long-term survival data to document the efficacy of neoadjuvant hormonal therapy for prostate cancer. However, the preliminary results suggest that it has merit as an emerging treatment option. The use of hormonal treatments for regional prostate cancer just prior to and during radiation treatments has been associated with improved control of the local tumor and reduces progression in the pelvis. A properly conducted, randomized study demonstrated that tumor stage was lower following hormonal treatments than it was for a similar group of patients who did not receive hormonal treatments beforehand. There has even been a small percentage of patients who had no cancer found in their prostate glands when a radical prostatectomy was performed following neoadjuvant hormonal treatment!

I recently heard from one such patient, who was diagnosed with stage B2 disease, combined Gleason score of 7, at age fifty-six. He first learned about neoadjuvant treatment by reading my article in *Scientific American* and decided to seek that treatment, which had not been discussed as an option by the physicians he consulted. He received a full year of neoadjuvant hormonal treatment followed by a radical prostatectomy. At prostatectomy there was no cancer found in his gland. He is very happy with his decision and his outcome and plans to publish a full account of his case, including his medical records, on two Internet newsgroups dedicated to the topic of prostate cancer (see Appendix). He is, he comments, "now a convinced and vocal missionary and advocate for neoadjuvant CHT [complete hormonal therapy]."

Most neoadjuvant therapies have utilized three months of hormonal treatments before a definitive procedure, such as surgery or radiation therapy, is performed. My own point of view is to provide at least six months of treatment. If the goal is to reduce the size of the primary tumor and to eradicate smaller micrometastatic deposits, a longer duration of treatment may be more advantageous, although by no means proven. A recommended program now used by many investigators relies on the PSA level to determine the length of treatment. The neoadjuvant treatment is provided until the PSA value reaches its lowest level and then for two months thereafter. For the majority of patients, this turns out about to be about six months.

You should bear in mind the fact that neoadjuvant hormonal therapy will reduce or eliminate your sexual activity for its duration. Not all men lose sexual interest and potency with short-term hormonal therapy. However, these men are exceptions, and you should not expect to be sexually active during neoadjuvant treatment, even if the shorter duration of three months is used.

If sexual activity is not an issue, then a course of hormonal treatments can be considered for men with stage B and or C cancers prior to definitive treatment with surgery or radiation. It is still a nonstandard treatment and is not widely available except in the context of a clinical trial. However, a number of specialists are providing neoadjuvant hormonal therapy for selected patients, following special investigational protocols developed by their institutions. As more and more information comes in, support in favor of neoadjuvant treatment to help control prostate cancer continues to increase. The challenge of obtaining access to this and other nonstandard treatment options is discussed again later in this chapter.

CRYOSURGERY

Cryosurgery uses the application of extreme cold to destroy abnormal tissue. It has been used successfully for some time to treat specific eye, skin, and gynecological abnormalities (for example, genital warts). Its application to deep-seated tissues or organs—such as the prostate gland—was technically difficult because these areas could not be directly visualized.

Beginning in the early 1990s, a number of refinements in cryosurgical devices and techniques were introduced that have made it possible to apply this modality to treating prostate cancer. TRUS technology now allows the cryosurgeon to visualize the prostate gland while inserting improved cryosurgical probes that use liquid nitrogen to deliver extreme cold to target tissues.

Cryosurgical treatment for prostate cancer is done under either a general anesthetic or local anesthesia (epidural block). The procedure generally takes about two hours, with about one and a half hours needed for inserting the probes and the remainder for the freezing procedure and removal of the probes. An ultrasound probe is first placed in the rectum to visualize the prostate gland. The surgeon then passes the probes through the perineum (the area between the bottom of the scrotum and the anus) into the prostate. Usually five probes are needed to "treat" an entire prostate gland—fewer if you have already had radiation therapy.

After probe placement, the super-cooled liquid nitrogen is allowed to flow into the probe's tip, delivering cell-killing temperatures to the gland. At the same time, the urethra must be prevented from freezing by introducing a warming solution via a catheter. Patients are able to leave the hospital within one to two days. They are generally followed up over the next few months and years, since it takes the body's defense mechanisms about nine to twelve months to scavenge and remove the dead cells.

To monitor the long-term effects of cryosurgery, repeat biopsies of the treated prostate gland are generally recommended at three months, one year, and two years after treatment. The positive biopsy rate is about 19 percent at two years following the procedure. Unlike radiation therapy (after which patients cannot be re-treated), cryosurgery patients can be treated with freezing again. This will often reduce the positive biopsy rate to 9 percent.

Cryosurgery is an attractive option to many patients who perceive it as less invasive and less risky than a radical prostatectomy. Unlike radical prostatectomy, external-beam radiation therapy, or interstitial radiotherapy, cryosurgery cannot be recommended with the same degree of confidence because the long-term data are not yet in. We don't yet know if it offers comparable success in eradicating local cancer, and many U.S. urologists view it as an inferior treatment modality, suspecting that it will prove to have a higher incidence of disease recurrence later on. Nevertheless, cryosurgery deserves mention as a potential treatment choice for selected individuals, with the full knowledge that the outcome and efficacy data are limited, compared to other treatment modalities.

Currently, there seem to be several schools of thought about which patients are ideal candidates for cryosurgery. A few physicians are using the cryosurgical procedure for patients who have previously received radiation therapy and are now found to have residual cancer in the area of the prostate gland. As discussed in Chapters 9 and 11, the recurrence of prostate cancer after radiation treatment is problematic to manage, and cryosurgery is now one possibility of dealing with local recurrence. It may prove to be a more acceptable alternative to "salvage" prostatectomy or hormonal therapy.

A second group of patients who are candidates for cryosurgery are those with suspected clinically localized disease, such as stage A, B, or certain stage C patients. Here, cryosurgery is competing head to head with more conventional surgery or radiation treatments. Some experts feel that if the gland is very large, cryosurgery may have limited value. Others suggest that neoadjuvant hormonal treatments can be used to shrink the gland prior to the cryosurgery. It is difficult to say who should consider cryosurgery and for what reasons, since the procedure is relatively new and only a few articles describing it have appeared in the medical journals.

Significant complications from cryosurgery include damage to the urethra. In rare cases, this damage may result in abnormal flow or leakage of urine, or blockage of urine passage through the urethra. Incontinence is reported in about

3 percent of cases. Prostatic infections can also occur. The standard complications associated with having any operation and with anesthesia are also possible with cryosurgery. The data concerning potency after cryosurgery are more difficult to assess because of the relatively short period of follow-up. Several physicians have reported that about 20 percent of patients who were potent before undergoing the procedure are potent at the six- or twelve-month follow-up. It is expected that more patients will report regaining their sexual function with longer-term follow-up.

As of late 1995, it was estimated by the manufacturer of the cryosurgical device that nearly six thousand prostate cancer patients have been treated with cryosurgery. The equipment needed to perform the procedure is currently available in about one hundred hospitals in the United States. Reimbursement policies for the procedure are not uniform. Many private insurers will pay the surgeon's and hospital costs, although there is no formal Medicare reimbursement at the time of this writing.

INVESTIGATIONAL TREATMENTS FOR ADVANCED DISEASE

Nonstandard and investigational treatments for metastatic disease are covered in Chapters 13 and 14 but are briefly introduced here, since they may have future applicability to patients with regionally advanced disease or cancer recurrence after treatment for localized disease.

Intermittent Androgen Blockage

Standard hormonal therapy, as described in Chapter 13, is continuous, and results in universal loss of sexual desire and ability. To improve quality of life for men with metastatic disease, a new approach is currently being evaluated to see whether intermittent hormonal therapy may be just as effective in controlling disease progression. In this approach, the hormonal therapy is delivered until the PSA value declines to a predetermined level. Then the treatment is stopped until the PSA rises again, allowing some men to recover their potency during the drug-free part of the cycle. In theory, this approach might prolong the time until the tumor becomes resistant or refractory to hormonal treatment.

Chemotherapy

Hormonal therapy is not a form of traditional cancer chemotherapy, as many patients initially believe. While hormonal therapy aims to cut off the supply of androgens that promote cancer growth, chemotherapy uses cytotoxic (toxic to cells) agents to destroy the cancer cells. Although chemotherapy is a standard treatment for many other types of metastatic cancer, such as cancer of the breast, its usefulness for the treatment of metastatic prostate cancer was never well established, especially since the older chemotherapy drugs were quite toxic and did not seem to offer advantages to hormonal treatment.

The chemotherapy drugs now being evaluated for use in the treatment of metastatic prostate cancer include estramustine, paclitaxel, vinblastine, adriamycin, and etoposide, usually in a combination therapy. At present, these agents are generally reserved for the treatment of hormonally resistant prostate cancer. If effective and less toxic chemotherapy approaches become available, they may be offered as an alternative to hormonal therapy, or even as a neoadjuvant or adjuvant treatment for men with locally advanced disease, but this is unlikely to be the case in the near future.

"DOCTOR, WHAT WOULD YOU DO
IF YOU WERE ME?"

Mr. Robert Bendler, fifty-three years old, illustrates the difficulties involved in recommending and providing non-standard treatments. For the past six years, his PSA had been in the range of 10–12, but evaluation by DRE and TRUS showed only BPH. After being treated for suspected prostatitis, his PSA was still elevated, but a biopsy again showed only BPH. In 1994, his urologist felt a change in the texture of the gland, prompting an additional biopsy. This time, the result was positive, with a Gleason score of 3 + 4. The diagnostic workup suggested a small, organ-confined cancer. However, when he came to our clinic, we also tested his blood-acid phosphatase level, as part of an investigational evaluation. It was elevated, raising the possibility that the cancer might be more extensive than a PSA level of 11 ng/ml would ordinarily suggest.

Mr. Bendler's referring urologist had suggested that he see someone at his hospital who was performing cryosurgery. This specialist recommended a protocol of nine months to one year of hormone treatments followed by cryosurgery. A second consulting urologist at a different institution called the cryosurgery recommendation preposterous, and recommended a radical prostatectomy (the non-nerve-sparing variety) with a simultaneous penile implant to manage postoperative impotence. Mr. Bendler felt that having both the prostatectomy and implant done at the same operative time made great sense, especially since the likelihood of maintaining potency was less than 50 percent.

When he came to our multidisciplinary clinic, our radiation therapist recommended a radical prostatectomy. Radiation treatments were not advisable because the patient had a long-standing history of prostatitis and urinary retention (inability to urinate). The surgeon who was seeing patients in the clinic also recommended a radical nonnerve-sparing prostatectomy.

I then saw Mr. Bendler and concurred with the diagnosis based on the findings seen on the various pathology slides, X-ray films, and physical examination. I was reluctant to recommend radiation treatments for the same reasons they were not recommended by the radiation oncologist. Both the patient and his wife had done a great deal of reading prior to our visit. In my conversation with them, I reviewed all the potential treatment options. These included watchful waiting, brachytherapy, cryotherapy, radiation therapy, and radical prostatectomy, either nerve or nonnerve-sparing variety. For the sake of completeness, I also mentioned the possibility of neoadjuvant hormonal therapy followed by either radiation treatments or radical prostatectomy. Mrs. Bendler was taking all this information down, adding it to her already full notebook of information and excerpts of consultations with other physicians.

Finally, Mr. Bendler asked me point-blank, "Doctor Garnick, exactly what would you do if you were sitting in my seat? Tell me how you would be treated." Although I had been asked this question many times before in one form or another, I usually did not answer it directly as posed. Instead, I tried to convince the patient that what I might choose might be best for me but not for him. Instead, what I could do was help him and his family look at the choices to arrive at the medical decision that made the most sense for his situation.

This time, I felt I did have a great deal in common with Mr. and Mrs. Bendler. He was only a few years older than I was, and I really could imagine myself sitting in his place, trying to decide what I would do. After several minutes of solemn thinking about my response to his question, I stated in no uncertain terms that if I were in his situation, I would opt for six months of hormonal therapy, in the form of an

LHRH analogue and an antiandrogen. I would then reassess my PSA, undergo an additional biopsy, and if positive, make a decision at that time to undergo a radical prostatectomy or, less likely, radiation therapy.

The idea of downstaging the tumor with hormonal therapy is an appealing one for me. A large percentage of patients will have positive margins at the time of radical prostatectomy and will require either radiation or hormonal treatments at some time in the future (in a so-called "salvage" situation). While the approach of neoadjuvant hormonal therapy followed by definitive local treatment is investigational, I would nonetheless select that treatment for myself; and since the question was posed in a way that required a direct, forthright answer, I had to provide it.

The ironic aspect of my response was that even though I would choose hormonal treatment followed by localized therapy, I could not readily offer it to Mr. Bendler, since it was an investigational treatment, and at that time our facility had no such clinical research underway. This was the most confusing information of all for the Bendlers.

"Well, where could I get such treatment if I wanted to?"

"There is a study being conducted in New York, where patients are receiving hormonal treatment before surgery. However, that particular study is a randomized study, so not all patients are going to receive the hormonal treatment before surgery. Only half will get the treatment, and that half is determined by a coin toss. Also, the length and type of hormonal treatment are not what I would opt for. They are using three months of hormonal treatments followed by surgery, and my suggestion is for a longer duration—six months."

By now Mrs. Bendler was getting angry. They had come to this high-powered academic institution for information and advice, and the treatment that they were advised about seemed to be unobtainable in its current form. Herein lies a

major problem. To adequately answer all the questions regarding the risks and survival benefits of a given treatment
may take more than a lifetime. Thus clinical judgment and
experience must enter into the evaluation of these promising but unproven treatments. The health-care bureaucracy
and the medical legal system can have a subtle or not-so-
subtle influence on prescribing an individual treatment that
is not considered "standard." Short of writing a clinical research proposal for approval by a peer scientific group and
risk-benefit evaluation by the institutional review board, I
would be unable to provide Mr. Bendler with this treatment
option, as it may not become a standard of care for five to
ten years. Thus, it is generally easier to recommend "standard" treatment, which in this case is radical prostatectomy,
and allow both him and you to get on with treatment.

Is Mr. Bendler being denied the best possible treatment?
Definitely not. Critics of my proposal will state that there is no
good evidence that the use of neoadjuvant hormonal therapy
will offer any advantage in terms of survival or other benefits.
(However, as mentioned, this seems to be changing.) Since
the long-term results of this treatment are not established, he
is not being deprived of any known benefits—except the potential wisdom and judgment of an individual who has very
strong convictions about what may prove to be right in the future. The discussion continued on the pros and cons of my
"recommendation for me" approach. As we left it, the patient
and his wife were going to give additional thought to how vigorously they wanted to pursue obtaining the "investigational"
approach that I had outlined. They later decided to take the
option of a radical prostatectomy with a penile implant, as discussed in Chapter 12.

Since Mr. Bendler was seen in our hospital clinic, we
have evaluated other patients whose risk of extracapsular
disease makes them potential candidates for neoadjuvant
hormonal therapy. A protocol is being developed to help

answer this very important question concerning the use and timing of hormonal treatments in patients with localized prostate cancer.

James Rainey, also fifty-three years old, was seen one week after Mr. Bendler. He had a PSA of 7.5 ng/ml, followed two months later with a repeat value of 7.8 ng/ml. A prostate gland biopsy revealed a Gleason 3 + 4 carcinoma with evidence of extensive disease throughout each of the six biopsy samples obtained. A nearly identical discussion to the one held with the Bendlers followed, with both the patient and his wife asking, "What would you do, doctor?" I recommended a six-month trial of neoadjuvant hormonal treatment followed by reevaluation, and then another decision regarding prostatectomy or radiation. We creatively worked out an arrangement with the patient's referring urologist where I would be advising the treatment program and would follow the patient during the period of hormonal treatments. The treating physician who gave the neoadjuvant treatment worked in a facility that had fewer restrictions about non-standard treatments than my facility. Also, the drugs (hormones) that are used for neoadjuvant treatments are commercially available for advanced prostate cancer even though they do not have a specific indication for neoadjuvant treatment.

ACCESS TO NONSTANDARD AND INVESTIGATIONAL THERAPIES: A QUICK ROAD MAP

Research continues to discover new applications for older therapies, new combinations of existing therapies, and, of course, new therapies. Assuming that you have learned about a nonstandard or investigational treatment and believe it may offer real benefits for you, how do you go about obtaining this treatment? Is it in fact available in your area, or at an institution you could consider traveling to? Will your insurer or HMO pay for it?

The problem is illustrated by Michael Malloy, a forty-nine-year-old sales representative. His medical circumstances are similar to Mr. Rainey's, but the manner in which his care is being rationed is worthy of comment. Mr. Malloy's father had been diagnosed with prostate cancer at the age of sixty-five. Because of this family history, Mr. Malloy had a PSA screening test that returned a value of 8.5 ng/ml. A surgical consult was obtained, followed by MRI and TRUS evaluations of the prostate gland. Both were unremarkable except for the presence of one suspicious area, which when biopsied showed a Gleason 3 + 4 carcinoma. The only symptom was the onset of impotence in the past year. The surgeon recommended a radical nonnerve-sparing prostatectomy with immediate penile implant.

Mr. Malloy sought my opinion after having had the consultation preapproved by his managed health-care board's "review" committee. He was seen by a urologist, a radiation oncologist, and myself, and again the question of "what would you do?" came up. The concept of neoadjuvant treatment was discussed and Mr. Malloy decided in favor of it. Because the managed health-care facility did not want to relinquish the patient's care to our facility, a series of calls between health-care providers ensued. Mr. Malloy wanted to transfer his care to me and the surgeon who saw him, but was unable to do so. I am now seeing and helping facilitate his neoadjuvant care with his primary-care physician (on my own time, without any charges to the managed-care organization). We are still working out the details of getting a surgeon of choice for Mr. Malloy, rather than the one assigned by the managed-care organization. The experience, a discouraging one for both Mr. Malloy and myself, suggests that as the pressure to control health-care utilization builds, access to nonstandard treatment options may become yet more difficult.

For investigational drugs, clinical trials of new treatments are often multicenter—meaning they involve physicians and patients at a number of locations—a design that helps eliminate the possibility that some local factors might influence treatment response or lack of response. You can learn whether any clinical trials are taking place in your area by accessing the National Cancer Institute's PDQ on-line computer program (part of CancerNet), or by calling NCI's Cancer Information Service at 1-800-4-CANCER. The Appendix gives fuller directions for finding this information.

However, as the Bendlers learned, clinical trials are normally randomized. A certain number of randomly selected individuals will receive the experimental treatment while the others will receive a standard treatment. Whenever possible and ethical, these trials are also "double-blind," meaning that neither the physicians nor the patients know who is getting the experimental treatment and who is getting a standard treatment. This is done so that the the investigator's and patient's hopes—powerful healing forces in their own right—do not skew the results in favor of the new treatment. Participation in such a trial is often the only possible access to a very new investigational treatment. Since all the patients in a clinical trial are monitored and followed with greater-than-average vigilance, there may be benefits for you to participate, even if you do not receive the investigational treatment.

For approaches that have passed through the first round of clinical investigation but are not yet considered "standard" and so are not generally available, individual physicians may be providing them to selected patients whom they believe would benefit, when the physician's institution—and/or the patient's insurer—agree that the treatment is medically valid. Oftentimes, it requires a very determined physician and an equally persistent patient to get those necessary blessings.

"IS THERE MORE THAT CAN BE DONE?"

In the next five to seven years there is likely to be more definitive information relating to the the risks and benefits of neoadjuvant treatments, cryosurgery, and other nonstandard therapies. What is the patient to do until then? The answer to this specific question and the more general issue of deciding upon treatment choices with inadequate information—awaiting studies that may be years in the coming—poses a dilemma for patient and physician alike, and can best be illustrated by the stories of two of my patients.

In the first case, that of Joe Papp, we now have the answer. The second case is taking place as you read this book. We will not know for some time whether the treatment decisions selected for Alfred Owens were correct or inappropriate. At least he had the ability to select his program with the most current information available at the time.

Mr. Papp, sixty-five years old, was found to have extensive prostate cancer involving his ribs, vertebral bones, and long bones of the lower legs. At the time of his diagnosis in the late 1980s, the standard treatment consisted of either undergoing a bilateral orchiectomy or receiving DES (diethylstilbestrol). As covered in Chapter 5, I and my colleagues at the TAP Pharmaceutical Corporation and investigators at the University of Utah and University of Colorado had recently demonstrated that the LHRH analogue leuprolide was as effective as DES, but with fewer side effects.

At this same time, the concept of using an LHRH analogue with an antiandrogen as a combination hormonal therapy was being discussed within investigative circles. Although prevailing opinion held that combining hormonal treatments added little or no benefit, preliminary data from investigators suggested that this combination might extend survival. At that time, however, gaining access to the anti-androgen flutamide required knowledge of the regulatory pathways, since it was still considered an investigational drug.

Mr. Papp did not want a surgical castration and also did not want to risk the cardiovascular complications of DES, since he had a history of hypertension (high blood pressure). He pinned his hopes on the yet-unproven combination treatment of the LHRH analogue plus the antiandrogen. Over the next four years, Mr. Papp's metastatic disease nearly completely disappeared. As would be the case with any treatment he selected which decreased the circulating levels of androgens, he was rendered impotent, lost his sex drive, and became less physically intimate with his wife. He accepted these losses gracefully because he was feeling so well and productive in all other respects. In fact, his emotional intimacy with his wife increased.

Then his cancer became resistant to the hormonal treatment, and in the last four months of his life, he suffered from the effects of advanced prostate cancer: agonizing bone pain, weight loss, muscle weakness, difficulty with walking, narcotic-induced constipation, and lethargy. He died fifty-four months after his initial diagnosis, having survived much longer than the eighteen to twenty-four months that would have been expected had he been given standard treatments.

Chances are excellent that the then-experimental treatment of the LHRH analogue plus the antiandrogen was responsible for his prolonged survival. This possibility raises the issue of whether all patients with incurable illnesses should have access to new, promising treatments which have not yet gone through the regulatory hurdles and may not be available for years—too late, perhaps, to provide them with meaningful benefits. The AIDS activists have increased awareness for the need to expedite availability of investigational therapies, and we are likely to see additional efforts for other difficult-to-treat diseases. Expanded access to investigational therapies continues to be hotly debated by physicians, pharmaceutical companies, regulatory authorities, and patient-advocacy groups.

In Mr. Papp's case, the encouraging preliminary data on the combination treatment were later supported. Based upon the initial National Cancer Institute study (discussed in Chapter 5), the FDA approved the therapy, and the combination-treatment approach is in wide use today. Yet, for every instance in which preliminary data are eventually confirmed, there is another where an initially exciting treatment proves useless or dangerous (such as high-dose DES). There is also the risk that giving patients early access to drugs will prevent clinicians from carrying out large trials in which patients are randomly chosen to receive either an experimental treatment or a standard therapy. Failure to perform these trials may hinder efforts to evaluate safety and efficacy. However, when people are dying and existing treatment strategies are inadequate, waiting for the perfect studies to be conducted is far from ideal. Some compromise must be devised in which regulatory agencies allow more flexibility, and pharmaceutical companies are encouraged to make investigational drugs available to patients who have life-threatening illnesses. For such a system to work, the federal agencies and the drug companies must be assured of continuous feedback about side effects and efficacy from the physician and the patient.

The second story, that of Alfred Owens, represents a different aspect of this problem. In his case, we are not dealing with the use of an investigational agent, but rather with the possible gains of applying existing treatment modalities in a new and unique fashion.

Mr. Owens was diagnosed with stage C prostate cancer at the age of sixty-nine. An elevated PSA exam and a CT scan showed involvement of the seminal vesicles, leading his physicians to recommend hormonal treatments, which were given. A recommendation for local treatment, such as radiation therapy or surgery, was not made. When he came to see me less than a year later, his prostate gland had shrunk remarkably, and he was otherwise well. The seminal vesicle involvement which was so prominent on his previous CT scan had all but disappeared on his current scan. There was also no other evidence of metastatic disease. All along, Mr. Owens had been told by his physicians that his disease was incurable, and that the hormonal treatments were the least invasive for him. He had resigned himself to a brief period of cancer remission followed by inevitable metastatic disease and death.

While this may indeed be the case, there is a possibility that he is curable. Unlikely, but possible. After a frank discussion, I recommended a course of radiation treatments to the local prostate gland with the idea that the hormonal treatments have shrunken and possibly sterilized his regional prostate cancer involvement (and possibly micrometastases). Consolidation treatment with radiation treatments may provide greater control and elimination of his primary cancer.

The idea of going for a cure gave Mr. Owens a completely different outlook. From being withdrawn and depressed about his situation because cure was never mentioned as a possibility, he had something to hope and to work for—which could only help.

The rationale for adding a local modality of treatment to a systemic one has its roots in the preliminary data regarding neoadjuvant treatment. Encouraging results suggest that the prostate gland can be substantially decreased in size, and one can hypothesize that smaller nests of cancerous cells may also be eliminated. I argue that it is worth the chance that more good is being done by adding the hormonal treatments to the radiation treatments, rather than waiting for evidence of metastatic disease, when the chances of cure are nil. When the treatment options are presented in this way, there are few patients who would not avail themselves of the chance to go for a cure. Oftentimes, narrow thinking pervades the physician-patient conversation, and the opportunity for creative problem-solving is missed. Maybe in the end skepticism will win out, but until that time emerges, my approach is to go for a cure if there is no evidence of documented metastatic disease.

Patients must continually question: "Is there more that can be done?" "What other modalities are available to me at this time and at my stage of disease?" "Are the risks worth taking, even though my physician and I know that the more aggressive treatments may not benefit and may actually result in some harm?" These questions need to be discussed, especially when the standard treatment is not expected to be curative, or cancer has recurred post-treatment. Providing hope, in and of itself, can be the most important and even most healing service a physician can offer to a patient. I was recently impressed by this very proactive attitude exhibited by Michael Milken on a recent Larry King show that discussed prostate cancer. Milken's unwavering attitude that questions and challenges the status quo is a very effective tool to increase knowledge, encourage the taking of risks, which will allow progress to be made.

11

POST-TREATMENT MONITORING

Today the PSA screening test is very often the first indicator that cancer my be present in the prostate gland. However, the usefulness of PSA testing is not confined to the initial screening and decision-making. After treatment, PSA monitoring is the primary tool for measuring treatment success and for detecting early signs of cancer recurrence. The PSA value and its velocity are valuable tools for assessing the need and the options for further treatment. You will continue to have regular PSA tests throughout life as an early-warning system to detect residual or recurrent disease. Let's not forget that a significant percentage of men with a normal PSA will have an abnormal DRE, and both should be done!

PSA LEVELS AFTER TREATMENT FOR LOCALIZED DISEASE

All the information about the normal range of values discussed previously is not relevant to the patient who has had definitive treatment for localized prostate cancer, either a radical prostatectomy or radiation. A man diagnosed with localized (stage A or B) cancer and treated surgically by radical prostatectomy should have his PSA level drop to undetectable levels (0 ng/ml) since the entire gland has been removed. A detectable level, even though it falls within the "normal range," in a postprostatectomy patient signifies the presence of residual prostate cancer. Neither the physician nor the patient should have a false sense of security if the PSA is 2 or 3 ng/ml. It means that the patient has residual or recurrent prostate cancer! Oftentimes, the PSA is the first harbinger of recurrent disease, even though it may predate any symptoms or clinical evidence of the disease by months or years.

For the patient treated with radiation, the evaluation is a bit more complex. Oftentimes the value does drop to zero. If, however, it is 1 or 2 ng/ml, it may be the case that some of the normal prostate tissue survived radiation treatment and is still producing PSA. If the value continues to rise, there is reason to be concerned that either cancer has spread outside the gland, or the radiation treatment did not eradicate the cancer within the gland. Very recent studies have shown that for optimal results, the PSA should be less than 1 ng/ml, and even less than 0.5 ng/ml. Levels that are above 1 or 2 ng/ml or greater twelve to eighteen months following completion of radiation treatments are very worrisome, since the cancer has not been eradicated.

Unlike the situation in which patients have an elevated PSA value following radical prostatectomy, patients who have been treated with radiation therapy are probably more likely to have residual rather than metastatic disease—cancer that was not eradicated by the treatment and survives in the prostate gland itself. The best management of these cases is not clear, particularly when the only evidence of disease is the elevated PSA. The physician's responsibility is to treat the patient, not the lab value, yet often the patients in this situation are too worried to accept an approach of watchful waiting.

Melvin Parks is a seventy-two-year-old retired African-American, who in 1987 had a diagnosis of a stage B1, Gleason 3 + 3 cancer. He opted for definitive radiation treatments, which were completed without complications. His initial PSA was 14 ng/ml, and reverted to normal several months after completing his radiation treatments. Approximately four years later, his PSA, which was in the 1–1.5 ng/ml range, started slowly creeping up. At the current time, his value is 7 ng/ml. He has been extensively evaluated with repeat abdominal CT scans, bone scans, TRUS, and physical exams, including a DRE. There is no evidence of detectable metastatic disease.

While there are several potential diagnostic and therapeutic interventions, which include biopsy of the prostatic fossa (the area in which the prostate gland is located), initiation of hormonal treatments, and cryosurgery, we have opted to "hold tight" and monitor the rate of the PSA rise. Is it possible that the slow and very modest rise in the PSA could be due to normal prostate tissue? This is very doubtful. However, given the slow rate of rise, it is possible that many additional years may pass before any active intervention is necessary for either local disease control, or disseminated disease management.

On rare occasions, an area of recurrence can be detected on rectal examination as the only evidence of recurrent or residual disease following radiation treatments. Under these circumstances, and in very special situations, a "salvage" radical prostatectomy may be an option. The experience with this procedure is limited, and should be attempted by only a few experienced surgeons, since the complication rates can be much more significant. As Dr. William Fair points out, the patient needs to be braver than the surgeon! This is a very difficult operation because the radiation treatments eliminate the "anatomic landmarks" that the surgeon depends upon to know where important nerves and blood vessels lie.

It is difficult to locate the normal planes of tissue to be dissected, and there is often a great deal of diffuse bleeding that is hard to control. Nonetheless, for the patient with a focal, anatomically limited recurrence, plus a reluctance to undergo long-term hormonal treatments, it may be a possibility. One current approach for patients who have developed recurrent or residual cancer after radiation therapy is to administer 3 to 6 months of hormonal therapy, and then consider a radical prostatectomy. Complications do occur, but may be minimized if the patient received 3D conformal radiation treatments in the past.

This course of action was not considered in Mr. Parks's case, since he had no clear-cut evidence of a localized recurrence. We will continue to monitor him for signs of progression. In all likelihood, he will elect to receive hormonal treatment, but in cases such as his, it is unclear how long the hormonal therapy should be continued. Prolonged hormonal therapy does result in loss of sexual desire and potency for the duration of the treatments. In addition, early, continuous therapy could possibly encourage the development of resistance to hormonal therapy in the surviving tumor cells, so a shorter course of therapy or intermittent hormonal therapy may be preferable in such a case.

MONITORING THE PATIENT WITH A "POSITIVE MARGIN"

Daniel Husik, a sixty-eight-year-old teacher, poses an all-too-common issue faced by large numbers of men treated surgically for localized prostate cancer. Mr. Husik was followed annually with a DRE. In 1988, a small "ridge" was noted by his physician. A PSA test was 6.4 ng/ml, and several months later, returned as 6.5 ng/ml. A biopsy showed a Gleason 3 + 3 score. All other staging evaluations were negative and a radical prostatectomy was scheduled. His postoperative course was noteworthy for two events. There was an excessive amount of bleeding postoperatively, requiring intensive care for a period of twenty-four hours after the operation; and there was a pathologic finding of a positive margin—in this case, microscopic cancer in the area of the *urethral anastomosis*—the part of the urethra that is cut and then reconnected during the prostatectomy.

This is one example of a so-called "positive margin." The borders or margins of the surgically removed gland can be positive for cancer in any one of several places and, when detected, poses a particular dilemma for treatment after the operation. The surgeon strives to structure the operation so that the cancer is contained within the boundaries of the prostate gland when it is removed. The problem with a positive margin is that even though the cancerous area is microscopic, it is found at the cut margin of the gland. This implies that on the margin that was not removed from the patient, additional cancer cells may lurk. Most experts agree that the patient with a positive margin is likely to have a recurrence of the cancer, but the big questions are:

1. When will such a recurrence take place?
2. Where in the body is the recurrence likely to occur—will the cancer recur as an extension of the localized disease, or will it have metastasized?
3. Can anything be done preemptively now (in the immediate postoperative period) to minimize the risk of a recurrence?
4. If something can be done, what should it be—postoperative radiation to the area of the positive margin? More surgical removal of the area containing the positive margin thought to be left in the patient? Hormonal treatments? Cryosurgery?
5. Can the PSA help guide us in these circumstances?

The likelihood that a recurrence will take place is very high. The recurrence may take three to eight years to show up clinically, that is, as disease that can be palpated on DRE or detected by diagnostic tests and scans. Unfortunately, there is no way of knowing if that recurrence is going to manifest itself in the area of the prostate gland, or in lymph nodes or bone. The location may be important in determining the type of treatment to be given. For example, if the recurrence is limited to a small area in the prostate region, a small field of radiation treatments may be offered. In certain circumstances, a small local recurrence in the prostate area years after the original surgery can be successfully treated with another surgical procedure. If, however, the cancer manifests itself as a recurrence in the bones with no evidence of recurrence in the prostate region, a systemic approach would be more appropriate, since the presence of the cancer in the bones or other distant site would be best treated by hormonal therapy.

Let's return to Mr. Husik as we untangle the answers to questions 3, 4, and 5. The management of the patient with a positive surgical margin has been debated for years. Some physicians advise observation only while others undertake active treatment interventions such as postoperative radiation treatments or systemic treatments with hormonal agents. Unfortunately, there is no convincing data to support the use of any of the active modalities; hence, many physicians would wait for the recurrence to manifest itself. By following the PSA value, we can get good assessment of whether a recurrence has taken place.

When the PSA rises following a radical prostatectomy, with or without a known positive margin, the general approach is to "restage" the patient with a DRE, an MRI, a bone scan, and an abdominal pelvic CT scan. An ultrasound exam may provide some useful information, especially if there is a discreet localized recurrence in the area of prior surgery in the prostate gland, but sometimes it is too insensitive to show anything.

If there is no definite area of recurrence yet the PSA is rising, as it was in Mr. Husik, there is generally a high level of anxiety on the patient's part for active intervention. In this particular case, we opted to treat the prostate bed (the area in the pelvis from which the prostate gland was removed) with doses of radiation therapy. While one could argue that the recurrence as manifested by the rising PSA may be coming from some other area, in this particular case, the PSA did return back to normal several months after the completion of the radiation treatments and has stayed down.

An alternative approach would have been to initiate treatment with hormonal therapy. The idea here is that a rising PSA in a postprostatectomy patient almost always means the persistence of prostate cancer cells, even though we can't detect them by conventional testing. Because the cells may be lurking anywhere in the body, systemic hormonal treatments have the best chance of eliminating them. However, in the otherwise asymptomatic patient in whom it has taken several years for the PSA to go from undetectable to a level of 1 or 2 ng/ml, hormonal therapy and its attendant side effects may be too intensive a treatment.

Oftentimes, patients with an elevated PSA without any abnormalities on restaging evaluation will be "watched" for something to happen. This could be in the form of a bone scan turning from negative to positive, or the demonstration on CT scan of a suspicious metastatic deposit. Another option is to biopsy the prostatic fossa (bed) even in the absence of palpable disease. If the biopsy is positive, the patient can receive radiation; if negative, systemic hormonal treatments can be considered, or the patient may opt to wait and get no active treatment. In the end, this treatment decision becomes a judgment call made with the joint participation of the physician, patient, and family members. It should be made after a full discussion of the various options, side effects, and other issues of quality of life.

For the patient who has regained or maintained his sexual activity after the operation, treatment with hormonal therapy is very likely to eliminate both sexual desire and performance. Radiation therapy following prostatectomy often decreases sexual activity if given after the operation, but less certainly or severely than hormonal therapy. Mr. Husik was indeed sexually active after the operation. When his PSA went up ever so slightly from 0 ng/ml after the operation to 1.3 ng/ml nearly four to five years later, he was just too uncomfortable with accepting a policy of observation. Even though all of his restaging studies were normal, we decided upon a program of radiation therapy. The treatment was remarkably well tolerated and did not interfere with any of his daily functions, including sexual relations with his wife. (This is unusual. Most men should not expect to be sexually active when radiation treatments follow prostatectomy.)

PSA MONITORING FOR MORE ADVANCED DISEASE

Alfred Owens is a seventy-year-old retired technician, who in October 1993 was found to have both an elevated PSA value of 55 ng/ml and an enlarged prostate gland. A prostate biopsy showed a Gleason pattern carcinoma of 4 + 3. On staging evaluation with abdominal–pelvic CT scan, enlargement of the seminal vesicles was suspected. In the view of his physicians, this suspected enlargement, coupled with both the physical appearance of the gland and the elevated PSA, was strong enough evidence of stage C disease. They recommended hormonal therapy and did not consider either radiation or surgery as options. Mr. Owens was placed on combination hormonal treatment with an LHRH analogue and an antiandrogen, which was tolerated well except for total loss of sexual activity.

When I consulted with Mr. Owens in July 1994, I found his prostate gland to be of normal size without any evidence of hardness or nodules. His PSA was less than 1 ng/ml, and a repeat CT scan demonstrated completely normal seminal vesicles. These findings led us to treat him with post-hormonal radiation therapy with the hope that the hormonal treatments may have eradicated micrometastatic disease and the prostate cancer within his gland. We would not have considered the addition of radiation treatments had the PSA still been markedly elevated.

Critics will argue that there is no evidence that the combination hormonal therapy plus the addition of radiation therapy is of any proven value. They are probably right, if you apply rigid standards of demonstrating such benefit with lengthy, well-controlled clinical studies. But patients who are seeing a physician today want from their physician (or should demand from their physician) what he or she thinks is the best possible treatment. To me, this means not only today's standard of treatment, but the most promising investigational therapies that may be the best treatment in the next few years. If the treatment decision recommended is not considered "standard," the patient, physician, and family must discuss the risk-benefit tradeoffs of choosing a promising but not yet firmly proven therapy, and the physician must address the ethical and regulatory concerns raised by giving "nonstandard" treatment.

Mr. Owens completed radiation treatments with only some mild discomfort with bowel movements but had none of the severe radiation-treatment side effects. His treatment program is currently at a crossroads. He has now completed his radiation treatments and has received nearly eighteen months of hormonal therapy. We do not know for how long such treatments should be prescribed in the absence of documented stage D disease. One approach may be to withdraw the hormonal treatments. We would continue to follow his PSA and strongly consider restarting the hormonal treatments as soon as there is evidence of a rise in the level. In this way, he may regain some of his sexual function and enjoy an improved quality of life.

Mr. Owens had been told that his disease was incurable. He may still have a recurrence, but he is doing much better than anyone predicted at the time of his diagnosis, and his prognosis, based on his clinical stage, may have been too gloomy. The hope is that the combination of modalities may have actually eradicated his prostate cancer or retarded its growth in such a fashion as to improve Mr. Owens' quality of life and his ultimate survival. This is the goal of our treatments. Any decision that I render to a patient has this as the driving force, even though all studies, with all the appropriate validations, have not yet been performed. This type of dialogue and joint decision-making is what I find my patients want!

12

Sexual Issues

The sexual complications of prostate cancer treatment are often major issues for the newly diagnosed man and his wife or significant other. Until recently, physicians and researchers showed relatively little interest in recognizing and responding to patients' concerns about the impact of the disease and its treatment on sexual function and self-image. Because of the changing nature of prostate cancer, with younger, sexually active patients now being diagnosed more often, more attention is being given to developing treatments with a lower risk of impotence, and to providing options to men who do not regain sexual functioning after treatment. It is now common for cancer centers to have specialized professionals who help counsel and treat sexual problems resulting from prostate cancer or prostate cancer treatment.

The fact that the medical establishment has in the past been ill-equipped to deal with issues of sexuality dates back to the typical patient who was diagnosed with prostate cancer in past decades. Usually a man in his seventies or eighties, he often had other coexisting diseases, along with significant symptoms from his prostate cancer, and so was assumed to be sexually inactive. Patients diagnosed in the 1990s fit a different profile. Nevertheless, there is still a shortage of suitably qualified health professionals to deal with many of these issues.

Only now are issues of psychosexual function being actively addressed in men with prostate cancer. New insights into the medical and anatomic reasons for sexual dysfunction are also helping to solve the clinical (rather than emotional) issues of sexual dysfunction. There is a greater degree of specialization to deal with male sexual problems following prostate cancer treatment. Urologists are now being trained in the management of impotence and in providing appropriate medical intervention to help couples deal with it. However, to my knowledge, there has been virtually no meaningful effort to deal with the sexual issues of the partners of men treated for prostate cancer.

Although the term "impotence" is often used to describe the general experience of sexual dysfunction (unsatisfactory sexual functioning or inability to function sexually), recent research suggests that the term "erectile dysfunction" may be more descriptive and meaningful. Impotence or erectile dysfunction is extremely common, though seldom discussed or acknowledged, among all men, not just those with prostate cancer. The fact that a detailed sexual history is often not obtained before prostate cancer treatment makes management of impotence after treatment more difficult.

Sexual dysfunction problems are incredibly common among men treated for prostate cancer. The prostate cancer itself can often contribute to erectile dysfunction before any treatment intervention is undertaken, if tumor growth presses on the nerves needed for an erection. In a recent Harris survey of prostate cancer patients and their physicians (commissioned by US TOO! International), over 75 percent of those treated for their disease reported experiencing impotence and 70 percent noticed a decline in their sex drive. All the therapies directed toward treating prostate cancer either alter the anatomy of the blood vessels and nerves responsible for adequate sexual functioning, or decrease the levels of male hormones, which are a prerequisite for sexual interest (libido) and sexual function. Thus, when all is said and done, it is probably more likely than not that there will be some measurable decrease in sexual functioning in most men undergoing treatment for prostate cancer.

When a younger man with a small organ-confined tumor is treated with either radiation therapy or nerve-sparing radical prostatectomy, there is a higher likelihood of keeping the sexual complications to a tolerable minimum. Unfortunately, for a large number of patients, some degree of reduced erectile function is going to be an inevitable consequence of localized treatment. For the vast majority (probably greater than 90 percent) of men treated with systemic hormonal therapy, both erectile dysfunction and loss of libido are consequences of the treatment. Attempts are now being made to lessen these side effects by designing hormonal agents that do not completely suppress the synthesis of male hormones, but this goal is still a long way off.

My bluntness in presenting this information is based upon years of experience with treating patients with hormonal therapy, all of whom lost their ability to have an erection adequate for vaginal penetration, as well as many consultations with men treated with radiation or surgery who experienced significant sexual dysfunction. I do not intend to be either insensitive or callous. Patients become angry and even despondent post-treatment if they have been given false assurances or unrealistic expectations about the likelihood of complications.

Although advanced prostate cancer will result in sexual dysfunction as well as urinary symptoms, this chapter focuses on sexual problems that arise directly or indirectly as a result of the cancer treatment. The case histories included here illustrate important points about coping with sexual dysfunction and seeking effective "rehabilitation" (the official term for learning new behavior and skills to recover a function) and management of the problem.

RESTORING SEXUAL FUNCTION: THE TREATMENTS AVAILABLE

There are three general types of treatment for sexual dysfunction following radical prostatectomy or radiation therapy. One form is called *pharmacological erection therapy* or PET therapy (also known as intracavernous vasoactive injection therapy). The second type of treatment utilizes a vacuum device which is able to inflate the penis by the use of suction. A third, surgical treatment involves the implantation of a penile prosthesis—such as a rod that make the penis semirigid.

Although there are other treatments available for impotence, they are generally not applicable for patients with erectile dysfunction resulting from prostate cancer treatments. For example, a man with diabetes might become impotent because of disease in the blood vessels required for erection, and specialized surgery can correct this specific problem. Such an approach is unlikely to be of benefit for the man with impotence following prostate cancer surgery.

In trying these different therapies, the best advice I can give you is simply to be patient. Because all of the treatments discussed in this section take some time to get accustomed to, you and your partner should not be discouraged if initial results are unsatisfactory or if it seems too unnatural or unspontaneous. Stick with it until you develop a certain level of skill or give it your best effort. On occasion, changing physicians may be necessary if the therapy provided doesn't work for you.

PET Therapy

While there are no absolute guidelines for choosing one treatment over another, most specialists will try PET therapy as the initial treatment for erectile dysfunction following a prostatectomy. With this technique, medicines that cause the penis to enlarge and become rigid are injected directly into the shaft of the penis before planned sexual intercourse. This is not more painful nor much more difficult than any other form of self-injection. It does take time to accept and learn the technique.

The patient has to be motivated to master this type of treatment, and must be evaluated medically to minimize the likelihood that an unexpected side effect will occur. In addition to changes in blood pressure, persistent erections (a condition called priapism) can occur, which requires antidotes to relax the penis. This type of injection therapy is much more likely to be successful if the patient and his partner are fully informed about the technical aspect of giving the injections. The physician who trains the patient in the injection therapy method must be compassionate and take the necessary time to explain the technique adequately. The lack of patience on the part of the physician is often one main reason for the patient to become discouraged and give up before developing the skill needed for this form of therapy.

There is still debate about the optimal drug or drug combination with PET therapy. Experts all recommend different medicines, with claims of fewer side effects and pain. The patient must realize that some experimenting will be required before the most satisfactory program is found. Any coexisting medical conditions, such as high blood pressure, may narrow down the choices. Possible medication interactions also have to be taken into account in selecting the correct PET therapy. The FDA just recently approved penile injections of a drug called prostaglandin for the management of impotence, under the brand name Caverject.

Advances continue to made in this treatment. For example, some of the medicines may now be administered directly into the urethra, using a suppository specifically made for this purpose. Although it is not yet clear how effective or dependable this method is in achieving an erection, the benefit of avoiding the injection is very attractive to patients. Urethral insertions of medicine may well become the treatment program of choice in years to come.

Yohimbine

Yet another potential pharmacological treatment for impotence is the drug called yohimbine. This drug has been available for nearly sixty years. Since it was introduced prior to the regulations imposed by the Food and Drug Act, it has never received formal approval by the FDA. In several studies yohimbine (sold as Yocon or Yohimex) has resulted in improved sexual function in nearly 50 percent of men with impotence due to psychological causes. Other studies have had less positive results. Its value in restoring sexual function in the patient with prostate cancer who has been treated with either radiation therapy or radical prostatectomy is not well established, although it may oftentimes be used. Its main side effects include dizziness, anxiety, nervousness, headache, and elevated blood pressure, but these effects are rare.

Vacuum-assisted Devices

The second type of treatment for erectile dysfunction uses a vacuum-assisted device. A cylinder is placed over the penis, then a vacuum is created with a pump, which in turn creates an erection. This is an attractive option for men who do not like using the injections and who do not want a surgical implant. Again, success requires a highly motivated patient (with good manual dexterity) and partner, as well as a compassionate and dedicated trainer.

The Penile Prosthesis

The third treatment involves the surgical implantation of a penile prosthesis. There are three forms of penile prostheses that are in use today—semirigid, malleable, and inflatable. A malleable prosthesis consists of two silicone rods that are permanently firm. However, they can be bent up for use during intercourse, and bent down, in a position closer to the body, when not used for sexual intercourse. The semirigid types are firm all the time, with less capacity for bending.

The inflatable type is a more complicated arrangement consisting of three major components—the penile cylinders that are implanted into the penis, a pump, and a reservoir. The pump is usually placed in the scrotum and when squeezed, causes the reservoir to push its fluid into the penile cylinders, causing an erection. The reservoir, which contains only about 100 ml (3 plus ounces) of fluid, is generally placed in the lower abdomen. The uncircumcised male may have to be circumcised as part of the placement of the cylinders into the penis.

Evaluations by patients generally indicate that between 70 percent and 80 percent are satisfied with a penile prosthesis. Reoperations to correct a mechanical malfunctioning are needed about 20 percent of the time. Infection occurs in 5 percent to 7 percent of patients, and generally is higher in patients with conditions such as diabetes or heart problems; erosion of the device through the skin occurs in less than 10 percent of patients. You should also know that the prostheses are usually made from silicone, a substance similar to the breast implants which have received so much media and legal attention. While the silicone has been reported to shed from the prosthesis and lodge in lymph nodes in the pelvic area, no significant silicone-related medical problems have resulted from the widespread use of these implant devices.

Because of the high incidence of impotence resulting from radical, nonnerve-sparing prostatectomy, a few surgeons will now implant a penile prosthesis at the time of the radical prostatectomy. In this instance, one urologist performs the radical prostatectomy. At the completion of this procedure, a second urologist enters the operating room and performs the second operation of implanting a penile prosthesis.

There are advantages and disadvantages to such an approach. For the sexually active patient who is going to be rendered impotent from the radical prostatectomy, combining both procedures accomplishes "one-stop shopping," bypassing the sometimes depressing trial-and-error process of trying the nonsurgical therapies. However, it eliminates the option of performing a nerve-sparing approach in the hopes of preserving potency, and it means you will never find out if either PET therapy or a vacuum-assisted device might have worked for you. While the implant is generally considered satisfactory by the men who choose it, there is a considerable reoperation rate to correct malfunctions as well as other shortcomings that keep the prosthesis from being the final answer for all patients.

One of my patients chose this option and is quite satisfied with the outcome. Robert Bendler, a fifty-three-year-old professional, had a PSA that stayed in the 10–12 ng/ml range for a number of years. The first biopsy found only benign enlargement and infection, but a later biopsy showed cancer. He chose to have a nonnerve-sparing surgery to maximize his chances for cure, and he had an inflatable penile implant done at the same time that included a pump placed in the scrotum.

I present this as one option which is appealing to many patients. In one prestigious Boston area hospital, the results of the "nerve-sparing" surgery have been so unsatisfactory that the surgical staff have abandoned the technique altogether. Their approach is to perform a classical nonnerve-sparing radical prostatectomy and then implant a penile prosthesis directly afterward. Thus the patient, when he consents to the operation, knows that the operation is going to make him impotent, and that this problem is going to be addressed immediately with the penile-prosthesis implantation. Many may argue with such an approach, and claim that the patient is agreeing to a known complication, with little done to avoid it. I also do not feel that this is the best or the one-size-fits-all solution, since some patients may regain sexual activity after the operation. And, in those that don't, alternatives to the surgical implantation of a penile prosthesis may be more satisfactory.

Some may have concerns that the decision for radical prostatectomy plus implant may be made too quickly when the patient and his partner are both overwhelmed with the news of the diagnosis. There is also so much happening at the time of radical prostatectomy. The necessity for banking blood for an autodonation, the anxiety about hearing the surgical findings, plus the efforts to reestablish urinary function all make this an extremely difficult time. Plainly, there is not enough discussion time for the patient and significant other to absorb all of the possibilities of sexual rehabilitation. One step at a time—get the cancer taken care of, get the urinary stream working properly, and then address the issues of sexual rehabilitation. However, many are extremely pleased with this approach. I have now had more direct experience with this strategy and am recommending it more frequently.

FINDING A TREATMENT THAT WORKS

Mr. Martin Gorman represents the good-news bad-news scenario in prostate cancer treatment. In my practice, we try to avoid this particular situation. However, I would guess he represents more of the typical situation and the type of outcome that patients can expect to have. He is a fifty-year-old man whose self-worth and self-esteem were based largely on his sexual conquests and potency. Having attended a series of all-male military academies, his main drive in life upon graduation was to make up for lost time by treating himself with women around the world.

He began to have a variety of prostatic infections, all quickly responding to antibiotic usage. However, on the third or fourth episode, his treating urologist opted to do a blind biopsy, despite the fact that his ultrasound and PSA tests were completely normal. Much to the surprise of all, the biopsy came back as positive for cancer, Gleason 3 + 3, in two of the samples, one from the left and one from the right lobe of the gland. (All of the other staging studies were negative or normal.)

After his initial panic and shock subsided, Mr. Gorman did his research and booked the first available date for the surgeon he wanted to perform a nerve-sparing prostatectomy. The operation went well, with no complications, and a unilateral nerve-sparing procedure was performed. Pathology of the resected prostate specimen returned a well-confined prostate cancer involving both lobes of the gland, with clear margins, and a final Gleason pattern score of 3 + 3.

Given his totally normal erectile functioning and sexual activity with his wife preoperatively, Mr. Gorman anxiously awaited the return of sexual functioning. Six months later, it was dead as a doornail. Twelve months later, the same thing. By this time, his mild incontinence was essentially under control, requiring him to wear a pad only intermittently. However, his distress over his impotence, despite great sexual desire, bothered him to the point that he started drinking again, lost interest in his career, and began to gain weight. He continued to hold on to the possibility that a small percentage of patients do regain some of their potency as late as eighteen months after the operation. Such was not the case for Mr. Gorman, however.

The urologist who operated upon him referred him to a subspecialist in sexual rehabilitation. For Mr. Gorman, it was decided that PET therapy would be the most beneficial treatment to restore sexual functioning. Although squeamish about injecting his penis with drugs, he had some early success, and with trial and error, some degree of expertise was achieved in performing the therapy. However, the further away he got from active discussion and continued training in the technique of injection therapy, the more alien it became for him to do.

A repeat visit to his sexual rehabilitation physician did nothing to rekindle his interest in making a firm commitment to try it again. He consulted me at this time, quite depressed, and I suggested another consult and gave him a choice of nationally recognized experts in the field of sexual rehabilitation. For whatever reason, the chemistry between this second subspecialist and the patient worked.

The physician had a different method of explanation and showed empathy and total commitment to solving the problem, especially given the fact that the injections had worked occasionally. All this gave Mr. Gorman renewed enthusiasm to try to resolve his sexual dysfunction problem, which was eroding his quality of life, diminishing his usual enthusiasm for life, family, and work. By changing the technique of injection and manipulating the drugs and dosages selected, a consistently good result was achieved.

What I learned from Mr. Gorman's experiences is the need for physicians and patients to keep on trying to solve the problems created by treatment complications. It is too often the case that the physician believes his or her responsibility is fully met once the best chance for a cure is provided. When complications such as incontinence or impotence persist and do not respond to the first round of rehabilitation efforts, it is not enough to tell the patient to just "accept it."

In rehabilitation, compassion and dedication seem to be far more critical than technique and expertise. The interest and time that the second specialist took represented to me the critical component for Mr. Gorman's satisfactory result. As he later told me, the two most significant events in his life were the news that his cancer was organ-confined, and the eventual return of satisfactory sexual functioning with pharmacologic treatments. He has fully recovered and is once again a contributing member of society, meeting his own requirements for self-worth and his many responsibilities in work, family, and community.

DOUBLE LIVES AND DIFFICULT SITUATIONS

When I first encountered Jack Wilkins, I thought that his particular case was unusual. However, shortly after seeing him, I encountered a very similar situation with another new patient, Stephen Fisher. I discussed these two with my colleagues, and to my surprise, I learned that nearly every physician I practice with has encountered similar patients. Mr. Wilkins is a sixty-two-year-old male who had a nodule found in his prostate gland on a routine physical examination by his internist. A biopsy demonstrated a Gleason $3 + 2$ prostate cancer coming from the nodule. His PSA was 4.3 ng/ml, and the remainder of the diagnostic workup was negative.

I took Mr. Wilkins' history in the presence of his wife, as I usually do. When we came to the issue of sexual activity, information I generally try to get from both partners, I was told that he had been impotent for several years, for unknown reasons. His wife was clearly upset at this situation, but accepting of it nonetheless. There were no more relevent de-

tails to the sexual history. They had never sought sexual rehabilitation counseling, but rather attributed his lack of performance to the aging process. Now, with the diagnosis of
prostate cancer in hand, there seemed to be an explanation
and vindication of the husband's impotence.

Before beginning the physical exam, I asked Mrs. Wilkins to wait in the reception area. As I started to examine
Mr. Wilkins, he pulled me aside and unabashedly whispered
that he was very much sexually active, and that he had been
having an extramarital affair for many years with a younger
woman whom he saw twice a week. This relationship was extremely important to him, and any decision about treatment
should be aimed at maximizing his chances for preserving
his sexual potency. His affair, I was told, was as important a
facet of his life as anything. Under no circumstances should
I mention his sexual activity to his wife, nor should there be
any mention of it in his medical record!

I found myself in a very compromised position. The
brochures I give to new patients and their spouses outline in
great detail the need for a frank discussion of side effects affecting sexual functioning, and how these complications can
be managed, and what the consequences are likely to be. After the physical exam, when the Wilkinses and I discussed
the various options, Mrs. Wilkins quite reasonably commented that if surgery was choice, then the radical prostatectomy should be done, given her husband's long-standing
impotence. She understood quite well that if you were impotent going into the operation, there was a zero chance of regaining potency following the operation. And so, she said, a
nerve-sparing procedure might increase the risk of leaving
behind cancer-containing tissue, with no appreciable benefit to be gained.

Her husband took the tack of "never say never," saying he
always had hopes that his potency would return some day.
Thus, he did not want to completely eliminate any chances of

that happening by undergoing a nonnerve-sparing operation. He was willing to hope for some return of potency, even
at the theoretical risk of leaving some cancer tissue behind.
We definitely did not solve this problem at this sitting. What
we did agree upon was the choice of surgery as the preferred
treatment. A referral was made to one of our surgeons, who
performed a pelvic lymph-node dissection (all were negative), followed by a unilateral nerve-sparing prostatectomy.

When the surgical staging was done, cancer was found in
both the right and left prostate lobes, and at the apex of the
gland. There was tumor present in the capsule, and some
nerve fibers in the prostate gland had been invaded with
cancer—together indicating a very high risk of recurrence.
Shortly after the operation, at about the four-month point,
Mr. Wilkins was able to have semifirm erections, completely
regained his sexual interest, and was once again sexually active. He had always thought that it was necessary to have a
fully rigid erection in order to have an orgasm. Much to his
delight, this was not the case, as he and his lover have re-
joiced on many a weekly occasion. However, from his wife's
perspective, the operation did nothing to help him regain
his erectile function.

While this story could have ended here, I selected it for
yet another reason. There is a great deal of debate regarding
postoperative treatment based upon the findings of capsular
penetration and cancer present at the apex of the gland. As
discussed in Chapter 11, the best treatment option for a "positive margin" is unknown. Had potency not been an issue,
many physicians would have opted to treat Mr. Wilkins in the
immediate postoperative period with either adjunctive radiation therapy or even hormonal treatments, since his risk of
cancer recurrence was quite high. This was not done, even
though it was offered to and refused by the patient.

Now, nearly three years later, his PSA, which had fallen to
undetectable levels initially, is rising. He is currently under-

going radiation treatments for his residual cancer, as measured by PSA. Whether the earlier initiation of this treatment would have delayed or prevented his PSA relapse is not known. What is important is that his sexual needs and interests were made a part of the decision-making process, though the decision never made sense to his wife, nor would make sense to anyone who did not know of Mr. Wilkins' "secret life."

Stephen Fisher, diagnosed with prostate cancer at age sixty-five, presents a very similar situation. He and his wife had not engaged in sexual relations for some years. A combination of some medical problems on her part, and lessened interest on his, were given as the reasons. Again, during the physical examination, he confided in me that he had been having an extramarital affair for the past few years, and wanted his treatments to maximize preservation of his potency. During the discussion of treatment options, Mr. Fisher was clearly opting for radiation treatments, somewhat to the surprise of his wife, who thought treatment with a radical prostatectomy would be preferable. Mr. Fisher was treated with radiation therapy, has done well, and has been able to maintain his potency now, several years after completion of his treatments.

13

HORMONAL TREATMENT FOR METASTATIC PROSTATE CANCER

This chapter examines the treatments available for state D metastatic prostate cancer—both early or D1 cancer, when the only evidence of metastases are the positive lymph nodes—and D2 cancer, where the bone scan is also positive and the patient may be experiencing pain. The standard first-line treatment for metastatic disease is hormonal therapy. Locally advanced stage C cancer is also frequently treated hormonally, often as an adjunctive or neoadjunctive treatment with radiation and sometimes surgery (see Chapter 10).

MANAGEMENT OF STAGE D1 DISEASE

The significance of stage D1 disease lies in the realization that the cancer is no longer confined to the prostate gland, but has spread beyond its confines. A policy of "watchful waiting" is often taken for stage D1 cancer, despite the fact that 80 percent of men with untreated stage D1 disease will develop evidence of stage D2 within a five-year time frame. When active treatment is selected for stage D1 disease, hormonal therapy is generally prescribed. We have good data (see Chapter 5) to support offering treatment early on, when there is a high expectation of improving both survival and quality of life.

Balanced against this reasoning are the issues of sexuality and potency. Nearly every hormonal treatment for prostate cancer which has as its main goal a reduction in the circulating levels of male hormones carries the side effect of loss of sexual desire (libido) and impotence. Thus, the decision to prescribe hormonal treatment is a sexually important one. The choice is between treatment now, with the hope that the tumor burden is less and more likely to respond to hormonal treatments, or treatment later, when the likelihood of developing stage D2 metastatic disease is greater and the treatments may be less effective.

My own view on this subject is to take a very detailed history from the patient. It is relatively unusual that the sexual drive is so demanding and important that patients opt for a delay of treatment. These individuals tend to be younger men, who may have more aggressive cancer. Here the delay is especially problematic, since one would want to initiate treatment sooner rather than later, given the evidence that prostate cancer may advance more rapidly in the younger patient.

There are several investigational options for the patient with metastatic disease who places a priority on maintaining his sexual activity. One of these is intermittent androgen blockade, described in Chapter 10—a treatment strategy in which "drug holidays" allow the patient to recover his sexual interest and functioning between periods of hormonal treatment. There has also been some research involving hormonal therapies that use the antiandrogen flutamide in combination with finasteride (Proscar) to limit the amount of DHT reaching the prostate without shutting down the body's synthesis of testosterone, which is needed for sexual potency. Whether the long-term survival benefits of these treatments will be satisfactory remains to be seen.

MANAGEMENT OF STAGE D2 DISEASE

Patients with bone metastases may have had metastatic disease at the time of initial diagnosis, or they may have developed it months or years after "localized" prostate cancer had been detected and treated. In the latter circumstance, it is more likely than not that the cancer cells eventually found in the bones were present even when the patient was being treated for localized cancer. The cancerous abnormalities, though, were too small to be detected by conventional means, and it was not until later that they grew to the point where they could be picked up by CT or bone scan.

There is no question about the need to institute treatment for these patients. There are a number of hormonal treatments available, with no universal agreement on which are to be preferred for which patients.

HORMONAL THERAPIES

Although hormonal therapy has long been established as the standard treatment for metastatic prostate cancer, uncertainties and controversies still exist. When should treatment be instituted? Are some forms of hormonal therapy more effective than others, in terms of improved quality of life, average survival time, or both? These questions are not likely to be finally answered any time soon, but once again, I will give you the information currently available, and then let you know my views and experiences.

To understand how hormones affect the prostate, I suggest you review the information in Chapter 5, which also describes the clinical trials that helped us arrive at our current treatment recommendations. Here I will only describe each treatment briefly, from the perspective of the patient considering his options.

DES

DES (diethylstilbestrol) is in one sense the "standard" for hormonal treatment for metastatic prostate cancer, since the FDA asks that researchers seeking approval for a new drug demonstrate its efficacy by comparison to DES. However, it has long been known that DES has significant cardiovascular side effects at moderate to higher doses. Physicians prescribing this drug sometimes try to limit the risk by using a dose of 1 mg, but at this low dose of DES, the testosterone level frequently begins to rise after six to twelve months of treatment. A dosage of about 3 mg provides better efficacy, though with increased risk of side effects. I do not consider DES a satisfactory option because of the risk of heart attack and other cardiovascular disease associated with it, yet it is still prescribed because it is inexpensive and relatively convenient to take as a daily oral pill. Some who prescribe DES advocate taking a "baby" aspirin daily to minimize the cardiovascular effects, but there are no studies to support this practice.

LHRH Analogues

The LHRH analogues, represented by leuprolide (Lupron) and goserlin (Zoladex), have been shown to be as effective as DES without the risk of serious cardiovascular side effects. They are administered as a monthly "depot" injection—which means it is formulated to release a continuous dose over a twenty-eight-to-thirty-day period. A new formulation will soon be available that requires only a quarterly (every three months) depot injection. The mechanism of action of the LHRH analogues is explained in Chapter 5. Given the side effects associated with DES, the LHRH analogues are, in my view, the drug of choice for metastatic prostate cancer, used as a single agent or (as described below) in combination therapy.

The LHRH analogues are known as *superagonists*, a term that refers to how they act on target receptors within the androgen synthesis pathway. The practical significance of this fact is that they cause a brief surge in testosterone production before they act to shut down testosterone production by the testes. A new class of LHRH analogues currently in development are LHRH *antagonists*. They may prove beneficial for patients who cannot receive leuprolide or goserlin because their disease is so extensive that the brief surge in testosterone caused by these LHRH analogues cannot be risked.

Bilateral Orchiectomy

A bilateral orchiectomy, or surgical castration, is sometimes recommended for an elderly man who cannot readily visit his doctor for a monthly injection of an LHRH analogue, and for whom the cardiovascular side effects of DES should not be risked. It may also be recommended if there is some concern that the patient will not be fully compliant with daily medication or monthly injections. If the patient does not feel the surgery will cause him psychological stress, it does avoid the costs and the inconvenience of the pharmaceutical alternatives. However, there is rarely a *medical* reason to prefer orchiectomy to the use of a drug. An exception would be a patient who has very extensive metastases and who requires an immediate shutdown of testosterone production. This was the case with Thomas DeMarco, described in the next chapter. However, it is more unusual today for patients to be diagnosed at such an advanced stage of disease progression.

Combination Therapy with an Antiandrogen

Orchiectomy, DES, and LHRH analogues all act to shut down the production of testosterone in the testes, as explained in Chapter 5. However, as much as 30 percent of the body's supply of the male hormones (androgens) are now believed to be produced in the adrenal glands. These androgens, which are closely related to testosterone, can also be converted to DHT and can promote prostate cancer growth. This raises the possibility that a second drug that shuts off this supply of androgens might have value in a combination treatment by achieving "total androgen blockade," also known as "complete hormonal treatment."

A class of agents known as antiandrogens act at the receptor level to prevent androgens from reaching the cell receptor and stimulating the cell to grow and divide. The antiandrogens are represented by the drug flutamide (Eulexin), which is taken orally as two capsules three times a day. These drugs have not been approved for use as a single agent (monotherapy) for prostate cancer. However, research has shown their value when used in combination with an LHRH analogue, or orchiectomy. In the NCI study described in Chapter 5, men with stage D prostate cancer receiving a combination therapy of leuprolide with flutamide enjoyed about a seven-month advantage in survival compared to patients receiving leuprolide alone. The advantage was nearly two years for patients with earlier metastatic disease. Some smaller studies did not show a survival advantage to the combination treatment, and other studies are underway to help decide the issue.

Until the advantages of combination therapy are established beyond question, some physicians, insurers, and healthcare administrators will feel that the costs and side effects of the treatment do not justify its use at this time. However, from a practical standpoint, it becomes difficult not to provide a stage D2 patient with the choice of receiving the antiandrogen in addition to an LHRH analogue. A potential seven-month survival advantage may not seem overwhelming to a policymaker examining the statistics, but it can be highly significant for the individual patient and his family!

Recent studies evaluating hormonal monotherapy in comparison to combined hormonal treatments have indicated that those patients with "minimal" metastatic disease are more likely to enjoy a prolonged survival with combination therapy, sometimes in excess of five years.

Side Effects

A word about the side effects of these treatments, since this, too, is an important component of any decision regarding treatment. Loss of sexual desire and impotence are the major side effects of any hormonal treatment that eliminates the body's supply of testosterone. Hot flashes and tenderness in the breast also occur to varying degrees with these therapies, although not every patient experiences them.

In patients who receive combination therapy, the incidence of diarrhea is slightly more common, due to the antiandrogen. While this problem is often self-limited, a rare patient may have to discontinue the antiandrogen because of the gastrointestinal effects. Likewise, abnormalities in liver function, resulting from damage to liver cells, are more apt to occur in patients receiving an antiandrogen and must be diligently watched for, especially during the early weeks and months of the treatment program. Failure to recognize this complication has on occasion been associated with irreversible liver damage and, in rare instances, death. You should not be concerned about the latter two (relatively remote) possibilities so long as you are being monitored with liver-function tests.

For the patient who already has kidney damage (hydronephrosis) or bone metastases from advanced disease, it is important to know that there is often a slight, transient worsening of the metastases when beginning treatment with an LHRH analogue. As explained above, this is because the drug increases the level of circulating androgens for several weeks before testosterone production is shut down. Combination therapy with an antiandrogen may avoid this effect. However, an LHRH analogue should not be used for patients with kidney blockage or metastases to the vertebrae because of the risk of a sudden worsening (exacerbation) of these conditions. The risk in the latter cases is that the tumor flare will put pressure on the spinal cord—an emergency condition when it occurs.

For this reason, for a patient with newly diagnosed metastatic prostate cancer which involves the vertebral bodies of the back (even if there are no symptoms such as pain or neurological damage), it may be reasonable to get a baseline CT scan or MRI of the back to be sure there is no tumor mass present which may possibly cause some cord damage. Spinal-cord compression is covered in greater detail in the next chapter.

COST SAVINGS AT THE PATIENT'S EXPENSE

You will remember reading about Dr. John Konrad in Chapter 4. His biopsy results were inadequately reviewed, and he himself did not return for follow-up because he believed the biopsy to be cancer-free. When he did visit his urologist a year and a half later, after his symptoms had worsened, he learned that he had prostate cancer. The biopsy showed a poorly differentiated prostatic adenocarcinoma, Gleason 4 + 4, in specimens from both the right and left lobes of the gland.

At this point, Dr. Konrad began to do research and to take an active role in his treatment decisions. He wanted to know the status of the lymph nodes that drain the prostate gland and whether they were involved with cancer cells. His urologist opted to perform a pelvic lymph-node dissection to make this determination. When I was reviewing his records, I was surprised that the surgery was done as the first resort, since he had not yet undergone an abdominal-pelvic CT scan. Dr. Konrad explained that he had asked his physician about the CT scan, especially as a means of looking at both the local extent of the primary prostate cancer and as an assessment of the draining lymph nodes. He was told that such a test did not have the resolution to evaluate the lymph nodes and was not ordered.

Nothing could be further from the truth, and I wondered whether it was a cost-saving measure in his managed-care system. There are numerous reasons for obtaining a CT scan. In addition to helping delineate the prostate gland and regional lymph nodes, it provides an assessment of the other organs within the abdomen, such as the liver. Most importantly, it provides an accurate assessment of the kidneys and ureters. Such an evaluation is especially important in the current case, since the reasons that brought Dr. Konrad back to his physician were the worsening of urinary symptoms, making an assessment of the urinary tract mandatory.

The pelvic lymph-node dissection had revealed that of sixteen excised lymph nodes, one of four nodes taken from the left side of the pelvis was positive for metastatic cancer, while none of twelve nodes removed from the right side contained cancer. The patient correctly diagnosed his condition as stage D1.

Dr. Konrad's bone-scan report had been read as negative. Yet our nuclear-medicine specialists (physicians who perform and interpret bone scans) felt that not only was the scan of marginal quality, but there were areas on the scan that could be interpreted as suspicious for the presence of metastatic disease. However, we had only a copy of the original scan. Additional evaluations, or better yet, another bone scan, had not yet been performed, making our assessment all the more difficult. This was a critical issue, since there was a significant possibility that Dr. Konrad had D2 disease, rather than D1.

The reason for giving these details relates to what you need to do in seeking a second consultation. In the current case, this patient had traveled a great distance to see me, and unfortunately, I could not provide the definitive answers he was seeking. If you are going to seek "second opinions," it is important to bring as much information as possible with you, including the original scans and X-ray reports. Often, the hospital bureaucracy will resist lending the original X-rays to the patient. You must persevere and demand them with the promise that they will be returned, since they will benefit you, the patient. When making an appointment for a consultation, it is also a good idea to ask what other diagnostic tests the consultant would like to have ordered, since it is often the case that opinions and treatment strategies cannot be offered until this information is in hand.

There we were with Dr. Konrad sitting in my office with newly diagnosed stage D1 prostate cancer. My evaluation was incomplete, mainly because I did not have access to a good-quality bone scan, nor did I have a CT scan with which to evaluate the abdominal and pelvic organs. The patient then told me that he had been placed on hormonal therapy in the form of 1 mg of diethylstilbestrol (DES) after he had been diagnosed with the positive lymph node. He said that his attending urologist felt that he definitely needed hormonal treatment, and that DES was as good as any other medication. Because DES had been written about extensively in the articles he had consulted, Dr. Konrad willingly, without vigorous questioning, started taking the medicine.

Why in 1994, would anyone prescribe DES when there are other medicines with fewer side effects and equal efficacy than DES? The simple answer is probably the pressure to reduce health-care costs, which may also have been the underlying reason for the errors of commission and omission earlier in this patient's history. Perhaps the urologist, pathologist, and the health-care administrators felt that even if Dr. Konrad had a well-differentiated prostate cancer a year and a half earlier, it was best left untreated, since he probably had the type of cancer that most people die with, rather than die of. How wrong and "costly" such thinking is!

Costs associated with differing treatments will always be considered in any decision. Critics will argue that the expense of various treatments does not justify the sometimes limited advantages, hence providing justification for third-party payers to reject claims for reimbursement. FDA approval of a costly drug provides strong justification for its use, and often the insurance company or other third-party payer will accept the claim without a fight. Nonetheless, it can be troublesome if a physician wants to prescribe the treatment for a patient whose profile does not exactly match the features that led to the drug approval in the first place.

In the initial leuprolide/flutamide study, the median duration of survival was approximately three years. If the cost of the medicine, in this case, the flutamide, is about $2,500 per year, this comes to approximately $7,500 for the three years of usage. One can determine the cost per year of life saved by dividing the seven months of extra survival resulting from the drug or 0.6 year into the $7,500 and come up with a figure of approximately $12,000 for a year of life saved. Comparisons with other types of therapies, such as dialysis, indicate that this is a very acceptable cost figure and can justify the use of these newer treatments.

THE PERSONAL COST OF CURE

Walter Kane, a fifty-six-year-old producer, had developed urinary frequency nearly eight years before seeking treatment. His evaluation showed an abnormally enlarged and hardened prostate gland, which on biopsy demonstrated a Gleason 3 + 4 cancer. His PSA was 12 ng/ml. His bone scan was normal, but on evaluation by CT scan, slightly enlarged lymph nodes in the pelvis were noted. A CT scan-directed biopsy of the lymph nodes, using needle aspiration, led to the diagnosis of "cancer cells present" in the lymph node, "compatible with a prostate origin." In other words, the cancer appeared to have metastasized outside the confines of the prostate gland and into the lymph nodes, making the diagnosis stage D1 disease.

Concerned about what to do, Mr. Kane urged that the most intensive and even investigational treatments be offered to him, since he did not like the overall statistics associated with stage D1 disease. At that time, we were in the process of developing an investigational treatment program which would treat stage D1 patients with systemic chemotherapy first, then offer hormonal treatments, with additional local treatment after completion of the chemotherapy and hormonal components.

In Mr. Kane's case, I treated him with intensive chemotherapy for three months, and then referred him to a radiation oncologist for external-beam radiation therapy to the gland. Upon completion of this second phase of his treatment, we then offered the patient an LHRH analog and the antiandrogen flutamide. The idea in this particular case, while totally speculative, was to maximize the anticancer effects of three differing modalities of treatment in a patient who was at extremely high risk of dying of his disease at some later point in time.

Survival, being there for his young grandchildren, was Mr. Kane's most important goal, at the cost of any suffering. We threw the book at him, trying every modality with an established track record for prostate cancer control—radiation therapy plus bilateral orchiectomy plus the antiandrogen flutamide. Treatments with a shakier record

of success for prostate cancer control, such as chemotherapy, were also given to this very concerned and informed patient.

The treatments were not without major side effects. During his hospitalizations for chemotherapy, the patient lost his
hair and became severely susceptible to infections because of
the chemotherapy's effects on the immune system. He also
developed some mild decrease in his kidney function as a result of the chemotherapy treatments. The radiation-therapy
treatments were fairly well tolerated, at least at the beginning, as was the total androgen blockade.

It is now nearly four years since his original diagnosis of
stage D1 prostate cancer, and Mr. Kane is alive and cancer
free! The statistics would have never predicted this. When
my colleagues, who criticized me for treating him so vigorously in the early stages of his disease, see him in my office
for his routine visit, they are quick to consider the possibility
that there is something to this very intensive multimodality
program. This may be a promising approach to consider in
selected patients, but longer-term outcomes will have to be
obtained before such treatments could ever be considered
routine.

However, Mr. Kane's quality of life has had a very rocky
course. He lost a great deal of weight, became depressed,
and developed urinary frequency and diarrhea as a complication of the radiation treatment. The urinary frequency in
effect disabled him from performing his day-to-day duties
in his line of work. Now on disability for nearly four years,
he is questioning his self-worth, since his treatments for his
illness have prevented him from working as a movie producer. He is concerned about how well his very understanding wife will continue to accept the situation for the
long term.

This particular patient makes me ponder whether we
are truly doing more good than harm in the vigorous man-

agement of our patients. Mr. Kane made it very clear that he wanted every modality to be given him, regardless of the cost in terms of suffering or quality of life. Because he was relatively young and had an excellent understanding of the side effects of all the treatments he elected, I agreed to try every available treatment strategy, standard or experimental. The fact that he is cancer-free is just short of miraculous, since the statistics would not have predicted this outcome. But the turmoil in his day-to-day life must be taking an incredible toll. When is the cure worse than the disease?

LONG-TERM SURVIVAL WITH METASTATIC DISEASE

Most, if not all patients, feel either consciously or subconsciously that the diagnosis of metastatic disease is synonymous with a death sentence. Statistics indicate that the median duration of survival (the time at which 50 percent of patients will have died) is between twenty-eight and thirty-six months for the stage D2 patient. However, you and your family must be aware that these are statistics only, and can never be applied to an individual patient.

Over the years, I have had the opportunity to care for patients with documented metastatic disease who have gone on to live ten to fifteen years or longer. Although there were not any common characteristics that would serve to identify these patients, the mere fact that such longevity is compatible with the diagnosis of metastatic prostate cancer is critical to realize. These patients, who numbered eight in all, were treated with different modalities, all had bone metastases, and for reasons that are still unknown, all had exquisitely sensitive cancers in terms of their response to either radiation or hormonal treatments.

While I do not honestly believe that patients with this kind of metastatic disease can be "cured," their prostate cancer can be well controlled to allow a nearly normal life expectancy. While this may not qualify as cure, it is the next best thing to it!

14

MANAGEMENT OF TREATMENT-RESISTANT METASTATIC DISEASE

The management of stage D3 prostate cancer, disease that is no longer controlled by hormonal treatments, is as complex and controversial as the management of early prostate cancer. Here, however, the numbers of treatment options are fewer, their effectiveness less, and an unsuccessful outcome generally means loss of life rather than loss of potency or continence. This is the time when critical decisions about priorities and treatment philosophy need to be established by the patient, his family, the treating physician, and other members of the health-care team.

Decisions about the management options for metastatic disease which no longer responds to standard hormonal treatments—hormonally resistant or refractory prostate cancer—should always take into account the patient's general health and level of functioning: his performance status. Performance status, briefly mentioned in Chapter 5, is the term applied to how well a patient is able to carry on normal activities of daily living. If the patient is able to work a full day or engage in normal daily activities unassisted, we say that he has a normal performance status, or a PS of "0" on one standard scale. On the other hand, a patient who is bedridden

100 percent of the time and cannot care for himself is considered to have a PS of 4.

The overall prognosis is closely correlated to the patient's performance status. Patients with a better performance status will generally tolerate treatments better and live longer than patients with a poorer performance status, when the reduced level of functioning is due to the underlying prostate cancer, not to other chronic medical conditions. It is obviously important to factor in any disability resulting from other medical conditions, even though the prostate cancer may not be contributing in a major way to that patient's disability. Remember the case of Samuel Taggert, whose lung disease was the major reason for his disability and the cause of his death.

CHEMOTHERAPY

Chemotherapy is still considered investigational in the management of prostate cancer. It may offer real benefits to patients with hormone-refractory disease who have a good performance status. However, it must be given in carefully monitored and controlled settings by physicians who are experts in administering chemotherapy in general, but who also understand the special considerations for giving chemotherapy to prostate cancer patients. These relate mainly to the fact that most men with metastatic prostate cancer have received prior radiation treatments that have affected their bone marrow, which makes it more difficult to tolerate chemotherapy's side effects.

Chemotherapy is the use of very potent chemical drugs that attempt to kill the cancer cells by interfering with the cell's ability to reproduce itself, or by causing chemical changes in the DNA of the cell to render it useless. Unfortunately, most chemotherapy is not selective for cancer cells.

The damage done to cancer cells is likely also to affect normal cells that are growing and multiplying rapidly. Depending on the chemotherapy used, tissues with a high rate of cell turnover will suffer some damage during the course of treatment. If, for example, the chemotherapy affects hair cells, then the patient is likely to go temporarily bald. Likewise, if the chemotherapy affects the lining of the mouth and/or the gastrointestinal tract, the patient may develop mouth sores, ulcers, or diarrhea. The most troublesome side effect associated with chemotherapy is a drop in white blood-cell counts resulting from damage to the cells of the bone marrow. When this occurs, a patient may be more susceptible to infections and complications resulting from infections. Damage to platelets, which are also formed in the bone marrow, may affect the blood's ability to clot, increasing the risk of bleeding complications. Nevertheless, chemotherapy may benefit an individual patient, in particular by decreasing pain from bone metastases.

SECOND-LINE HORMONAL THERAPY

Occasionally patients whose disease has become refractory to our standard hormonal therapies, described in Chapter 13, will obtain some relief from the so-called "second-line" hormonal treatments. These include aminoglutethimide and mesgesterol (Megace), ketaconazole, prednisone, and estramustine (Emcyt), which is a combination of an estrogen and nitrogen mustard, a chemotherapy agent. Second-line hormonal treatments are ones that have shown some effectiveness in controlled studies, but the results obtained are not seen as superior to DES, LHRH analogues, orchiectomy, or combined hormonal therapy with an antiandrogen. They are generally better tolerated than chemotherapy, but for the hormonally refractory patient, the benefit is often subjective (pain relief) without sustained objective signs that the disease has been controlled again.

INVESTIGATIONAL DRUGS

Oftentimes, a patient will be offered a totally investigational drug when his prostate cancer has become resistant to hormonal treatments. These investigational treatment programs are usually highly regulated and under strict scrutiny by hospital human-protection boards and government agencies and also by pharmaceutical companies, if they are overseeing the clinical investigation of a new drug for the treatment of prostate cancer.

There are several drugs that have emerged from treatment programs just described. A drug known as suramin, which was used many years ago for different reasons, has recently been shown to have some anticancer activity in patients with resistant prostate cancer. Although there may be very toxic side effects, the use of sophisticated means of dosing the drug seems to have cut down on the side effects.

It is also important to remember that drugs that are effective for the treatment of prostate cancer may not yet be approved for use in the United States, but may be available either in Europe or Canada. As explained in the Appendix and in Chapter 10, resources are available to find out what the latest information is on these drugs, and the criteria for being admitted to an investigational-drug treatment program. It may mean an occasional trip to the sponsoring hospital where the program is being done. If that is impractical from either a logistical or financial standpoint, there are generally ways to work within the investigational-drug network to obtain access to promising drugs.

DETECTING AND TREATING
SPINAL CORD COMPRESSION

While the selection of an investigational agent for the patient with hormonally refractory prostate cancer is an important decision, the actual day-to-day management of the patient is an even more important issue. Pain management is covered in the next chapter. Mild or moderate pain can generally be alleviated with non-narcotic analgesics, such as Tylenol, Advil, or Bufferin. If and when you have a new onset of back pain, however, you need to bring it to your doctor's attention immediately, to evaluate any risk of damaging the spinal cord.

As you remember, prostate cancer often metastasizes to the skeletal bones, including the vertebral bones that surround the spinal cord. If there is a cancerous deposit in one of the vertebrae, and there is any associated tissue swelling around that deposit, the tumor mass and swelling can encroach on the spinal cord and cause it to be compressed. When this happens, the blood supply that normally nourishes the spinal cord tissues is cut off, and there may be damage to the cord because of the reduced blood supply. If untreated, this condition can lead to paralysis of the lower extremities, or loss of bowel and bladder function. This is called a "spinal-cord compression" or for short, "cord compression."

If this happens, it is a medical emergency and requires immediate attention in the emergency room by a team of highly experienced physicians, including an oncologist, a radiotherapist, a neurosurgeon, and a neuroradiologist. Under no circumstances should you delay seeking treatment for even twenty-four hours if you have a new onset of back pain accompanied by symptoms of numbness and weakness in the extremities. The reason for the immediate attention is the possibility that some of the damage to the spinal cord can be reversed if the pressure and the swelling are relieved.

Studies have shown that the earlier the relief of pressure, the greater the likelihood is for recovery.

In one large cancer center, the most common reason for acute cord compression was metastatic prostate cancer. It generally occurs in a patient with known bone metastases to the vertebral column. There is either gradually increasing pain, or loss of function (such as weakness) in the leg, or difficulty knowing when you have to move your bowels or bladder. To diagnose cord compression, patients undergo a neurological examination. If this indicates muscle weakness, abnormal reflexes and sensations, or other types of abnormalities, damage to the spinal cord should be suspected. This needs to be further evaluated by X-rays of the vertebral bones and the spinal cord itself.

We have made great advances in diagnosing cord compression. Ten to fifteen years ago, the most accurate method for determining if a tumor mass was pressing on the spinal cord was an X-ray procedure called a myelogram. This painful, often dreaded test required the injection of "dye" (a substance introduced by a lumbar puncture or "spinal tap" used to surround the spinal cord) and then multiple twistings and turnings of the patient on an X-ray table to get appropriate pictures. Today, however, we can visualize the spinal cord easily by performing a specialized CT scan, called a spinal CT, or by doing an MRI of the spinal cord. Both of these tests are painless and highly accurate in pinpointing the exact location of the tumor so it can be treated.

If cord compression is suspected in a patient with known prostate cancer who is resistant to hormonal treatments (Stage D3), the first step is to administer very high doses of a cortisone-like steroid, usually dexamethasone (Decadron). The steroid helps shrink the swelling which may be causing the abnormal neurological functioning. An X-ray is usually then done to establish the diagnosis. If the cord compression is caused by a tumor, then one of two treatments is given, in addition to keeping the patient on the dexamethasone. The tumor mass can be removed surgically by a neurosurgeon or a specialized orthopedic surgeon, or the cancerous mass can be irradiated. Generally, the latter modality is selected because the ability of the neurosurgeon to get a good surgical result is lessened by the presence of cancer deposits in surrounding areas.

Thomas DeMarco is a fifty-two-year-old mechanic who came to his physician with new onset back pain and weakness in the left leg. The back pain had been present for about one to two weeks, but the weakness and difficulty in walking was more sudden, occurring over the past thirty-six hours. He had never had a diagnosis of prostate cancer, nor had he ever been screened. The neurological examination found a possible abnormality of the nerves from the spinal cord which control leg function. An immediate CT scan of this area of the back (this was prior to the widespread availability of MRI) showed an abnormality suggestive of cancer pressing down on the spinal cord. The DRE found a lump in Mr. DeMarco's prostate gland, very suggestive of a cancer.

Because the weakness in his leg was getting worse, an emergency call was made to our neurosurgeon, who immediately scheduled the patient for surgery. He had been started on dexamethasone, the surgical team was assembled in a matter of twenty to thirty minutes, and an operation was performed which removed the lump from the spinal cord. The analysis of the lump of the pathologist showed a cancer, compatible with a cancer of prostate gland origin. Indeed, his prostate gland was also biopsied, which confirmed the presence of the cancer there, as suspected by the physical exam.

The only choice of treatment for Mr. DeMarco at this time (in addition to the dexamethasone and neurosurgical procedure) was to do an immediate bilateral orchiectomy.

An LHRH analogue, such as leuprolide, was not warranted because it would take several weeks for it to work in lowering the body's level of male hormones. Although there were other investigational drugs that could be used, time was of the essence, and so an orchiectomy was performed at once.

The most remarkable aspect of Mr. DeMarco's case was his continued recovery of leg strength over the next three days and the resolution of his bone pain in the back. He went on to do extremely well, living with metastatic disease for several more years prior to developing additional bone metastases which required both hormonal and radiation treatments.

Mr. DeMarco is remarkable for several reasons. Unlike the majority of patients who develop spinal cord compression with stage D3 prostate cancer, his cord compression predated the diagnosis of his prostate cancer. This occurs but is quite rare. More importantly, the cord compression was quickly and successfully identified and treated. This makes the difference between a patient requiring nursing-home care (because of paralysis and lack of control over bowel and bladder function) and a patient who is self-sufficient! All too often, the diagnosis of cord compression is made too late, when irreversible damage to the nerves of the spinal cord has occurred.

The last reason for telling about Mr. DeMarco relates to the fact that any new back pain and new onset of weakness in the legs or arms demands urgent attention. Mr. DeMarco was lucky. Had he waited to seek medical attention, or had his physicians not acted so promptly, he could have ended up as a wheelchair-bound invalid for the rest of his life. You have got to seek urgent attention if any of these situations arise, especially if you know that you have prostate cancer, and that the cancer has lost some of its responsiveness to hormonal treatments.

MAKING THE TREATMENT DECISION

Philip Attager exemplifies the patient with hormonally resistant prostate cancer. Diagnosed at the age of fifty-one, Mr. Attager was found to have positive lymph nodes in both his pelvis and abdominal area. He was staged as having D2 cancer, rather than D1, because of lymph-node metastases found higher up in his abdomen.

He was initially treated with a single LHRH analogue, leuprolide, which promptly took his elevated PSA value to undetectable limits, where it remained for several years. When his PSA started to rise, a repeat CT scan, which had shown shrinkage of his lymph nodes with the hormonal therapy, again demonstrated enlargement, indicative of residual metastatic disease. His bone scan, too, had become positive.

At that point a second-line hormonal treatment was added to his program. This treatment yielded an initial decrease on the PSA for nearly seven to eight months. The PSA value then rose, along with some worsening of the bone scan. For the first time, he was mildly symptomatic, requiring some mild pain killers to relieve his pain.

Mr. Attager, who was now fifty-four, wanted to get the most promising investigational treatments available for what was now hormonally refractory prostate cancer. After a full discussion of the options, Mr. Attager decided to visit the National Institutes of Health to learn more about suramin, which had recently been shown to have beneficial activity in hormonally refractory prostate cancer. Although he could have obtained the drug through a program based in Bethesda, he decided not to pursue the treatment because of the side-effects profile described to him. He opted for a treatment program using an investigational hormonal agent and a chemotherapeutic agent.

The program could be administered from a hospital close to his home. He underwent the treatment, and was able to carry on his life reasonably well, until the last two months of his life, in which he was bedridden, with pain, loss of appetite, and progressive bone metastases. Radiation treatments were administered to several painful bony areas, which helped temporarily. From the time his disease became refractory and began to progress, Mr. Attager experienced a relatively rapid downhill course.

Mr. Attager had decided to seek out the available investigational-treatment programs because he wanted to give additional treatment a fighting chance, even though he understood the probability of arresting the disease's progression was low. The investigational program he selected was what he wanted because it did not require traveling to the sponsoring institution, had tolerable side effects, and allowed him to carry on his day-to-day routine until very near the end of his life. Others in a similar situation may have opted for the potentially more toxic suramin, or for nothing at all.

There is no right or wrong to these decisions. Mr. Attager made the decision that made the most sense to him—preserving his hope by trying another treatment while minimizing the side effects and the disruption to his daily life. He made his decision in consultation with me, with the support of family and friends, and all involved in his care were in agreement about the risks and benefits of the course chosen. Thoughtful optimism and a determination to do the most possible, never giving up, are psychologically important for the patient and family, and for the physicians.

There are situations where the patient or his family want one type of treatment, and the physician feels differently. Kenneth Young was seventy-two years old when he was diagnosed with prostate cancer. Although he had one suspicious area on his bone scan, his PSA was quite low. It was elected to treat his local disease with radiation therapy. About six months later, his PSA started to rise, and the previously suspicious area on bone scan was now more intense, suggesting disease activity.

Mr. Young wanted everything done that could possibly be done, and he was offered the choice between leuprolide and flutamide or orchiectomy and flutamide. He chose the latter, and at the time of orchiectomy, he had two testicular prostheses implanted, because he was very concerned with his body image. This treatment resulted in an excellent response both in his abnormal bone scan and the PSA elevation, which came back to a value of less than 1 ng/ml.

However, his PSA gradually started to creep upward, with some additional intensity in the original area of bone scan. He was, however, without pain from the bony metastases. Although my treatment philosophy is not to treat the older, hormonally refractory patient who has other medical conditions (he had both heart disease and some mild diabetes as well as another type of cancer), his family insisted that he have radiation to that one bone area, which was reluctantly performed.

Although this treatment was associated with a transient decline in the PSA value, it shortly thereafter started to rise. He was still asymptomatic, but because of the rising PSA, the family again demanded that additional treatment be given. I was extremely reluctant to treat the patient now. After all, I would be treating an elevated lab value, not a patient suffering from symptoms that needed to be alleviated. I did, however, agree to place him on some additional mild hormonal treatments, knowing full well that the likelihood of a response was extremely low. When his PSA continued to rise even more rapidly, they sought the opinion of another specialist, who was willing to place him on yet another form of reasonably well-tolerated hormonal therapy. Again, I was concerned about treating an asymptomatic and now seventy-six-year-old man with agents that were likely to make him feel worse than he was currently feeling, with little to gain on the other end, except for a possible fall of a few points in the PSA. This led to a conversation with Mr. Young and his family in which I explained why I felt uncomfortable in continuing to provide ongoing medical advice. We mutually agreed that it was in the patient's best interest to continue to be cared for by a physician who shared a very active treatment philosophy.

In my twenty-five years of practicing medicine, my inability to convince a patient that my recommendations were in his best interest has happened, fortunately, only a few times. This case was particularly difficult for me. Whether I should have acquiesced more is debatable. I had to convince myself that Mr. Young's interests were being fulfilled. I knew that I could not fulfill them by remaining on as his physician.

BEYOND STANDARD TREATMENTS AND CONVENTIONAL WISDOM

Joseph Papp was one of the most remarkable men I have ever had the pleasure of knowing. I can use his name freely, as his biographer Helen Epstein has already chronicled intimate details of his medical treatment in her recently acclaimed biography, *Joseph Papp: An American Story*. It is noteworthy that nearly every major review of this book discussed his medical condition and the impact this disease had on his life and on those who surrounded him at the New York Shakespeare Festival and the Public Theater. His story raises several important issues that are of significance to others facing the realities of metastatic prostate cancer.

In April 1987, when Mr. Papp was sixty-five years old, he had just been diagnosed in New York City by fine needle aspirate of having prostate cancer. His subsequent staging workup demonstrated a markedly positive bone scan with metastatic involvement of nearly every rib and many long bones of the extremities, as well as many bones of the vertebral spine. His PSA was nearly 200 ng/ml; his acid phosphatase was nearly 20 (with normal being less than 1), yet he was relatively asymptomatic and otherwise fully ambulatory and active.

For a variety of reasons, he sought medical treatment under my supervision in Boston. When I first met Mr. Papp and his wife, Gail Merrifield Papp, they had already done an exhaustive medical search on the various treatments available for patients with prostate cancer, and came in with a four-hundred-page computer printout compiled from the National Library of Medicine in Bethesda. I have always viewed this as responsible and desirable behavior on a patient's part. In the decision-making process for any complex-to-treat disease, an informed patient and family member can best assess the personal implications of the options. Discussing all the possibilities thoroughly does a great deal in make everyone feel aligned and part of the team whose goal is to beat the disease.

The results of Mr. Papp's tests showed extensive metastatic prostate cancer, a situation which demanded urgent treatment. Yet the results of the "standard treatments" were not overly promising for his stage of disease. The Papps wanted anything that was even the least bit more promising to be administered to Joe. At this time, the National Cancer Institute was evaluating the benefits of a combined hormonal therapy using an LHRH analogue with an antiandrogen. (This research is described in Chapter 5.) Although the results of the study had not yet been published, preliminary reports suggested that the combined treatments might be of more benefit than the LHRH analogue alone. The combination also had an acceptable side-effect profile, so that the treatment, while still unproven, was of low risk.

I felt that the new treatment was eventually going to be proven better than conventional treatments, and upon hearing of the preliminary data, the Papps opted for the experimental treatment. Although I had no direct access to the investigational antiandrogen which was part of the program, I knew the correct regulatory maneuvers to obtain the experimental treatment, was able to identify a source rapidly, and worked with my institution's Human Protection Board, the pharmaceutical sponsor of the drug, and the FDA to gain access and approval to use the drug in several days.

Mr. Papp's response to the treatments was nothing short of miraculous. His bone scan, which had been riddled with cancerous deposits, resolved to almost normal within the first six months of treatment. His PSA, markedly elevated at the outset, became undetectable with one to two months of treatment. Mr. Papp was able to resume his normally frenetic pace of life, globetrotting all over the world to further the cause of the New York Shakespeare Festival and to receive numerous awards and honors for his charitable and artistic achievements.

To me, his story illustrates two very important points that deserve comment, one generally referable to medicine and to the physician/patient relationship, the other specific to prostate cancer. There are tremendous uncertainties in medicine. To wait for the final answer is oftentimes impractical, and more than likely it is unobtainable. Thus, when a patient visits a physician, it is important for mutual respect and honesty to take precedence over ambiguities of yet-to-be-answered questions. Too often, physicians are paralyzed by indecision based upon inadequate information. We must overcome this to serve our patients well. In Mr. Papp's case, I thought the best treatment for him was the combination treatment, despite lacking the definitive answers. While I am not convinced that the investigational treatment was the sole cause for the remarkable response that his cancer showed to treatment, it was certainly a factor.

The second important point relates to the predictive

value the PSA has in the setting of metastatic disease. A rapid and sustained fall in the PSA value is a very promising sign that the cancer may be in remission for a long period of time. Studies have shown that a sustained fall to the normal range within one month of starting treatment is associated with an excellent long-term outlook. In contrast, when the PSA value does not decline to a normal level, or it does so only to rise again within a short period of time, the patient often will not enjoy a long-term or favorable remission status.

In Joe Papp's case, these teachings are borne out. His PSA fell rapidly and it continued to be normal or at undetectable levels for nearly four years of remission. His quality of life was essentially unimpaired during this time, except for his sexuality. His response was so remarkable that when he was in nearly complete remission, we even thought about trying to maintain and increase the likelihood of prolonging his remission by using other investigational treatments. Could we try to kill off additional cancer cells that we knew were lurking, but had not yet been identified by X-ray studies or by clinical symptoms? There was absolutely no information to suggest that we could ever "cure" Mr. Papp of his metastatic prostate cancer. While we were joyous that he had such an excellent response to his treatment, I knew that it could not last indefinitely.

Since radiation treatments are often used to control metastatic prostate cancer which has spread to the bones, we considered radiating Mr. Papp with either whole or hemibody radiation treatments to try and eliminate the microscopic cancerous cells in his bones. This treatment would involve the delivery of radiation doses to the entire body, in contrast to treating only a localized area of prostate cancer which had spread to the bone. Such a suggestion would be deemed preposterous by other specialists treating the disease. Yet I was able to tentatively convince one of my radiation-therapy colleagues to evaluate Mr. Papp for this consideration.

All the plans were made in advance for a consultation to take place between Mr. Papp and my colleague, who practiced at a prestigious academic institution. As is normally the case, the resident or physician took the initial medical history and physical examination before the "Chief" saw the patient. The resident was apparently so astonished by the reason for the consultation that he argued the Chief out of his tentative agreement to try whole-body or hemibody radiation treatments.

The Papps were led to believe that they were seeing the radiation specialist to initiate treatments. There was a breakdown in communication when the radiation oncologist stated that he considered that the radiation treatments had no merit, and that the whole plan should be aborted. My best attempts to try and think "out of the box" creatively had been thwarted, with some undermining of the Papps's confidence in me and my judgment. Fortunately, my relationship with Mr. Papp had been so solid that it was able to withstand this jolt.

The significance of this part of the story would only become apparent years later. Mr. Papp's disease had first reappeared in his left hip and eventually became so painful that radiation treatments were required to control the pain. Multiple areas of bone involvement were eventually found, and they were also treated with radiation. The cancer never returned in any of the areas where the bone was irradiated. On the left hip, metastatic disease eventually cropped up in all the surrounding bone, but it never reappeared in the well-circumscribed field that had received the initial radiation treatments.

That raised the eerie possibility that had we initiated treatment to all of the bones when Mr. Papp was in remission, we might have been able to delay the emergence of the metastatic disease which eventually claimed his life. We will never know the answer. His story again shows that creative thinking must be used in conjunction with traditional clinical practices when medical situations are life-threatening.

15

QUALITY-OF-LIFE ISSUES FOR ADVANCED DISEASE

This year about 318,000 men will be diagnosed with prostate cancer. And this year about 41,000 men will die of prostate cancer. Some will die of cancer that went undiagnosed or untreated until already far advanced. Others have had localized treatment intended to be curative, suffered a recurrence of cancer some years later, received hormonal treatments for months or years, and finally developed extensive metastases that were refractory to all existing treatments. This chapter offers information and guidelines for men and their families who are confronting the possibility, or the certainty, of dying of prostate cancer.

Throughout this book, I have expressed my belief in vigorous treatment, have rejected watchful waiting in all but a few exceptions, and have generally tended to consider investigational and novel treatments before all the scientific and medical data have matured. This philosophy carries through to the treatment of advanced, treatment-refractory disease, except that I pay more attention to issues of quality of life at this juncture, when treatment benefits do not always outweigh treatment side effects.

In the late stages of advanced disease, when the conventional methods of treatment have done their job and the cancer has now become refractory to them, there is only a small likelihood that an experimental agent will stop or slow cancer progression to any meaningful extent. Balanced against this possibility is the side-effect profile associated with the experimental treatment. In most cases, the patient has had prolonged hormonal therapy and probably radiation or surgery as well, and the cumulative effects may cause any additional treatment to be less well tolerated. Usually, too, he is an older man by this time and may have developed other medical problems.

My own treatment recommendations for advanced, refractory disease factor all of these items into the equation, with more emphasis placed on the patient's quality of life. To me, it is not worth administering a treatment that may prolong life by a week or a month if that time is spent coping with severe side effects. Because understanding and evaluating these tradeoffs is so imperative, new statistical methods are being developed to quantify the balance between competing outcomes—quantity of life and quality of life with and without treatment, or with different treatments. These statistical approaches are used to help the patient and physician predict the consequences of various decisions. These seemingly cold, but hopefully accurate numbers provide a rational, objective basis for making the highly personal and subjective decision about what matters most to you as your options and your hopes are diminishing.

WHAT PATIENTS WANT TO KNOW AND NEED TO KNOW

The issue of succession planning must be given consideration in the patient with refractory, metastatic disease. This can be one of the most sensitive areas to discuss openly and frankly. In great part, the case with which such a discussion takes place depends upon who initiates the conversation. Patients will be very explicit in their communications with physicians and with their family members. A patient who wants to know the score in terms of how much life is left, or what the probabilities are that any new modality will work, and if not, what then, will clearly communicate the need for this information. I have found that the patient will wait until he is ready to bring up such conversations. If a patient is actively involved in a business, where his death is going to have a material effect on the operation of the business, the patient himself or a family member would benefit from a discussion, in general terms, about life expectancy, realizing that no one has definite answers.

Patients themselves are generally very exact in obtaining both the type and depth of information they need when they realize that they face limited treatment options and the approaching end of their life. However, not all patients with advanced disease want to address the question of what they should expect in terms of pain or quality of life as their cancer continues to progress. A compassionate physician who had known the patient with prostate cancer throughout his illness can sense the appropriate timing for these discussions, whether with the patient himself or a close family member or significant other.

Early in my medical training, I remember watching as a man dying of metastatic prostate cancer made his will in the hospital room. That particular patient was the CEO of a very large corporation. I was confused about why such a prominent man would have waited to that point in his life to think about wills, estates, and succession planning. Now, many years later, I am no longer surprised, since such planning more often than not happens when advanced disease is present, driving the confrontation with one's own mortality.

I constantly think back on that experience when I am counseling terminally ill patients about their options. Physicians see it as part of their duty of fully informing the patient to tell him when it is time to make certain his affairs are in order because the prognosis is poor. In giving this information, physicians must above all be compassionate, caring, and optimistic, yet not misleading.

A very difficult situation occurs when the patient does not want to discuss, under any circumstances, estate planning and succession choices. I remember one case when I needed to seek the help of a colleague to help care for one of my patients. My colleague felt that it was his obligation to tell the patient about his advanced stage of refractory prostate cancer, the limitations of treatment choices, and that "his business should be put in order." At that point, he was not ready to either hear such news or cope with it. He never saw that physician again, and made it abundantly clear that discussions of that sort were not to happen unless he brought them up. His wife, too, respected this decision. At the time we all knew he was dying, but the discussion never surfaced. To hear it from me would have been so emotionally devastating and hurtful that I never formally addressed it. When I tell this story to my colleagues, I am often criticized for not having the frank discussion of death and dying with the patient and family. My judgment argued otherwise. I could not take hope away from this patient, which he and his family were able to maintain until the very end. The few inconveniences of estate planning which would have been best served by a discussion before his death were overshadowed by a continued positive attitude on his and his wife's part during the last two months of life.

PAIN CONTROL

Back pain, especially new back pain, is a problem that should be reported to your physician immediately, since the possibility of spinal cord compression, discussed in Chapter 14, must be evaluated and promptly treated if present.

The management of pain is often the central concern in advanced disease and requires the coordinated efforts of a multidisciplinary health-care team, the family, and the patient himself. Just as creativity and persistence are needed in seeking cure or control of cancer in the treatment-responsive stages, so the patient and the physician should explore all the available options to relieve pain and maintain quality of life at the best level achievable.

The pain of advanced prostate cancer usually results from metastases to the skeleton. Bone pain that is present in the patient with newly diagnosed metastatic cancer is generally very responsive to treatment with hormonal therapy. As we have learned, the prostate cancer cells are fueled by male hormones, and the removal of the male hormones by any one of a large variety of means is likely to shut off the growth nutrients to both the primary prostate cancer and the metastatic areas, causing cancer-cell death, but rarely eradicating the cancer. When this happens, patients like Thomas DeMarco (discussed in Chapter 14) who are diagnosed after seeking medical attention for pain will usually be relieved of it. However, once this initial treatment response to hormonal therapy has been achieved, the pain will eventually recur and is less readily treated.

Radiation Treatment

Often, if the pain is localized to a well-defined area in the skeleton and is no longer controlled by mild analgesics, it can be successfully treated with spot radiation therapy. In this procedure, a small field of radiation is applied to the abnormal bone which is causing the pain. Most often, the series of treatments will alleviate the pain. Problems arise if the bony area is located near the spinal cord or a vital organ.

The amount of radiation given has to be reduced, as there are limits to the amount the other tissues can safely withstand. Also, if additional pain develops at some later date, the use of radiation may be limited by virtue of the previous doses which have been given.

When a patient has become hormonally refractory and has widespread metastases in bones that cannot be safely treated with "spot" radiation, the patient and physician face a more difficult challenge. Under these circumstances, the pain can often be relieved with radioactive substances which accumulate in the diseased bone and deliver a dose of radiation to that specific area. One such radioactive compound is called strontium, which is given through the vein. It is taken up by areas of bone that are undergoing rapid repair or growth, which includes the cancerous areas. The cancer cells in those areas will die, providing a high likelihood of some pain relief. The results, when this therapy is effective, can be quite dramatic. The response is relatively short-lived, however, and repeated dosing may be limited by damage to the immune-system cells that are produced in the bone marrow, which also take up strontium.

Narcotics and Other Analgesics

When pain persists despite the use of spot radiation or the use of strontium, and the pain is no longer responsive to mild pain medicines, stronger analgesic agents are prescribed, usually narcotics. Every physician or specialist in pain control usually has a specific program that will produce a predictable degree of pain relief. However, I cannot emphasize enough the importance of continually reevaluating the pain program on a regular basis. Is adequate pain relief being achieved? What is the side-effect profile that is associated with the use of these particular pain medicines? How are these side effects being managed, and are they being managed adequately? If the physician is not actively addressing these questions, then you, the patient, or you, the family member, must bring them up.

It is extremely important for both the physician and patient to recognize that addiction is almost never a problem with these types of narcotic pain-control programs. The need for increasing doses to control pain should not be confused with drug abuse. In my twenty-plus years of caring for patients with metastatic prostate cancer, I have never seen one of these patients abuse pain medicines. A fear or perception of addiction, on the part of physician, patient, or family, may lead to underdosing, leaving the patient in a state of constant pain. Pain relief is the goal, and unless it is achieved, the physician has not performed his or her job satisfactorily.

Managing Constipation

While addiction is rarely an issue for a patient with bone metastases who requires pain relief, the side effect of severe constipation can be a very worrisome problem. Narcotic pain relievers have a number of effects on the gastrointestinal tract that contribute to constipation. They reduce the normal motility or motion of the bowels, and the patient may not be well enough or have enough muscular strength to force a bowel movement. When this happens, the fecal material or stool becomes hardened with a consistency similar to hard gravel or cement. This leads to a mechanical plugging of the lower rectum, making it virtually impossible for a patient to have a normal bowel movement. This condition is called a fecal impaction, and can be one of the most troublesome, yet overlooked aspects of patient management.

When I first met Michael Sheplee, he was considered to have widespread metastatic, hormonally refractory prostate cancer with many bony metastases. Pain was a significant complaint, and he had been taking narcotic painkillers, such as Dilaudid, Tylenol with codeine, Percodan, and Percocet in various combinations to control the pain. This pain-control program allowed him to take care of various business responsibilities and function at a moderate level.

Mr. Sheplee came to my attention one Friday afternoon as I was providing coverage for the chief physician's patients. He had abdominal pain and bloating, and reported that he had not passed any bowel material for at least six days. The physical examination revealed impacted (dried and hardened) fecal material in his rectum. I then proceeded to disimpact him—meaning I extracted the cementlike stool from the rectum bit by bit, using my gloved fingers, until only softer fecal material was left, which he could then eliminate himself. He then had a massive bowel movement (six days worth, in fact). The relief he experienced was so immense that I marked that moment as one of my more memorable in providing relief for a suffering patient. Believe me, it was not a high-tech maneuver, but a humanitarian act that is performed every day by nursing staff and often goes unappreciated.

Mr. Sheplee's experience underscores the importance of expecting this side effect when increasing doses of narcotics are being prescribed. The simple knowledge that constipation is a troublesome side effect of narcotic-pain medicines should prompt the patient and family to set up a prevention program of high-fiber foods, bulk laxatives, and other laxatives as needed. If the patient is eating normally, and normally has a bowel movement every day or two, then that should be the goal, even though it may require bulk laxatives and enemas.

Constipation can be overlooked by the physician yet be the most troubling problem to the patient, to the point that having a bowel movement is the most important event of the week. I cannot emphasize enough the importance and significance of this problem, which with a little planning can be avoided!

Other Pain-Control Programs

A coordinated team effort by pain-management specialists, anesthesiologists, neurosurgeons, social workers, oncology nurses, and nutritionists can provide very sophisticated and individualized interventions to improve quality of life when specific anticancer modalities have lost effectiveness.

Although not widely accepted as uniformly effective, the application of a transdermal electrical nerve stimulator (TENS) can be helpful in controlling pain for some patients. Small needles or electrodes are placed into the skin and then stimulated by a pulsing electric current. The patient can control the level of stimulation, which aims to disrupt the continual pain stimulus by stimulating another area, "distracting" the brain and the body's pain-awareness mechanisms. Even though the results of large studies have not shown TENS to have overall effectiveness, I have had several patients who have been able to decrease the amount of pain medicine required when a TENS device was added to their program of pain control.

Other pain-control approaches can target the specific site of pain. Specialists in anesthesiology can provide nerve blocks, in which specific nerves are injected with analgesics, decreasing the pain in the area of the body supplied by these nerves. This is a very useful treatment modality if the pain is in an area where the responsible nerve fibers can be identified and injected. This approach provides the added benefit of treating only the affected area, without using drugs that affect the entire body, including the brain.

Other sophisticated means of treating pain include techniques in which the patient determines his level of pain control by using external pumps containing the analgesic. By pushing a button, he can dose himself with the amount needed to control the pain. The pain medicine, usually morphine, is administered into the spinal canal, where it is more effective than it would be if taken orally or by intramuscular injection. Another delivery system uses a pump that is implanted in the body, usually under the abdominal wall. The pump containing the pain-killing medicine is hooked up to a small tube, called a catheter (but different from the urinary catheter used after a radical prostatectomy), which is placed into the spinal canal. Small doses of morphine are continuously "pumped" into the spinal area, which can provide significant pain relief and even get the patient back to a more normal lifestyle.

The patient who finds himself requiring these sophisticated pain-control measures has generally advanced to the stage of disease progression where very little benefit can be expected from either current or developing investigational treatments. The goal under these circumstances is *palliation*, or the control of pain and suffering. Patients will have symptoms that require specific intervention and the goal is to relieve those symptoms.

HELPLESSNESS AND DEPRESSION

As the cancer progresses and the patient becomes more weak and dependent on others, this helplessness often creates more distress than pain or the thought of death. The patient experiences a loss of control over his life and his body. Men who reach this stage of disease progression have generally lost weight, have difficulties carrying out daily self-care activities, and become very dependent on spouse, significant other, or family for their care. Privately, and in group sessions, they express their fear of being abandoned.

Others do not have a family member who can provide

the assistance they need as they become more and more dependent. The patient may be on his own, or living with an elderly wife who may have medical problems of her own. The couple may be overwhelmed with the tasks of caring for each other, which may become physically impossible. Financial burdens or the fear of a financial catastrophe oftentimes force decisions that do not provide the optimal solution to either the patient's or the family's needs.

A compassionate and knowledgeable social worker can provide great help in these circumstances. The social worker is the most qualified person on the team to help the patient and family look at ways of bearing the costs of nursing care and evaluating the possibilities for home versus institutionalized care. Even more, the social worker can help all involved cope with their individual burdens of guilt, anger, frustration, and grief—feelings they may not be able to share with each other. Diane Blum, Executive Director of Cancer Care, Inc., has done a great deal to advance psychosocial care for and sensitivity to the needs of prostate cancer patients and their families. The specialist social worker is becoming an increasingly important provider of psychosocial care for those with advanced prostate cancer, and also for men at earlier stages of the disease, when they are wrestling with decisions about treatments and complications.

HOSPICE CARE AND SHARED DECISION-MAKING

Alan Quint's story exemplifies what can be done to keep the final decline and dying comfortable, dignified, and meaningful when the patient, family, significant others, and health-care team all work together to provide the best quality of life in the last months of life.

Diagnosed when he was fifty-four, Mr. Quint had metastatic disease which was treated with an LHRH analogue for nearly three years before a rising PSA indicated recurrent cancer. Divorced years earlier and now with grown children, Mr. Quint was involved in one very intense, though long-distance relationship during the first two years following his diagnosis of prostate cancer. From my perspective as Mr. Quint's physician, I saw that Pamela truly loved him, and the warmth and tenderness of the new relationship, which was formed without sexual intimacy, was touching for me to witness. While there could be no sexual culmination, since his disease had left him impotent, there was a vibrant physical intimacy when Mr. Quint and his "lover" were together. The relationship ended, according to Pamela, because Mr. Quint felt so much self-pity and did not want to burden his lover with his medical problems. She, in a very strong fashion, wanted only to be by his side. He rejected these offers because he wanted to spare her that misery. Since they lived far apart and Mr. Quint did not accept her offer to be with him, the relationship gradually eroded.

Later on, Mr. Quint developed a close relationship with one of his health-care providers, Denise. She was significantly younger than he was, and provided a level of medical/technical involvement qualitatively different from his former partner. A marriage was even contemplated, but that idea was abandoned when his disease became both more progressive and symptomatic. His desire to spare Denise a painful involvement with him again eventually lessened their intimacy. However, she was more aware as a professional of what she would be getting herself into, and did not offer the same unlimited commitment that Pamela had.

Symptomatic bone metastases grew more problematic to manage. A family conference was held, which included Mr. Quint's children, Denise, a social worker, myself, a local physician close to Mr. Quint's home, and a hospice administrator. Putting Mr. Quint's wishes first and foremost, a plan was worked out that allowed Mr. Quint to stay at home with the support of his family and the health-care team, who together eased his pain and allowed him the dignity of self-care as far as his abilities allowed.

Even during this time, Mr. Quint expressed a desire to undergo investigational treatment with chemotherapy, as described in Chapter 14. A "can-do" attitude was imperative in allowing Mr. Quint to be in control of his life, to enjoy the meaningful involvement of all who loved him, to pursue his personal interests, and to stay in familiar surroundings until he died several months later. Hospice care can be a great contributor to quality of life for patients with terminal prostate cancer by providing essential care within the home. For patients whose medical problems are most significant, or whose family cannot provide the intensive support needed, an inpatient hospice setting is another option that can be considered, with the input and guidance of the social worker.

GLOSSARY

Abdominal-pelvic CT scan A computed tomography (X-ray) scan that examines the organs of the abdomen and pelvis.

Acid phosphatase A substance secreted by prostate-gland cells, both normal and cancerous ones.

Acid phosphatase test A blood test sometimes used to help determine the presence of metastatic prostate cancer. If elevated above the normal value, spread of the cancer beyond the prostate gland is suspected.

Adenocarcinoma A type of cancer, arising from specific tissues that form glands. Nearly all prostate cancers are adenocarcinomas.

Adrenal gland A pair of organs that are located above the kidney and that synthesize a number of important hormones, including adrenaline, androgens (in the male), and steroids such as cortisol.

Age-specific reference range (PSA) The normal values of PSA correlated to the age of the patient.

Analgesic A medicine or other treatment that relieves pain.

Anaplastic A more severe form of poorly differentiated cancer.

Androgens   The male hormones. Generally, androgens refer to testosterone and dihydrotestosterone (DHT).

Anemia   A condition in which there is a low or inadequate amount of red blood cells. Red blood cells function to carry oxygen throughout the body; consequences of anemia include fatigue and shortness of breath.

Antiandrogen   A type of drug that blocks the growth-promoting influence of androgens on prostate gland and prostate cancer cells.

Aspiration biopsy   A biopsy procedure in which tissue contents or cellular contents are pulled through a syringe.

Assay   A test or method for measuring a substance, usually in minute quantities.

Asymptomatic   The absence of specific complaints or symptoms, such as pain or fatigue.

Autodonation of blood   A procedure whereby a patient donates his own blood for use at a later time, usually during future surgery.

Benign   The absence of cancer, usually used of a growth or tumor; opposite of malignant.

Benign prostatic hyperplasia (BPH)   Enlargement of the prostate gland, usually accompanied by aging. It may be associated with an elevated PSA, but there is no cancer present in the gland.

Biopsy   A procedure for obtaining samples of tissue to determine the presence or absence of disease or cancer. It can be done using a needle or as a surgical procedure.

Bladder   The muscular sac that collects and stores urine made by the kidneys until it can be eliminated from the body.

Blind biopsy   A biopsy in which the needle for obtaining tissue is placed into tissue where there are no specific abnormal areas to guide the procedure.

Blood clot   An accumulation of the solid components of blood, located in a blood vessel. It is a dangerous condition, especially if the clot travels and lodges in another portion of the body, such as the lung.

Bloodstream The circulation of blood, which flows in blood vessels (arteries and veins) and bathes and nourishes all body organs. Substances (such as PSA and testosterone) may be made in one portion of the body and circulate in the bloodstream.

Blood-thinning agents Medicines that decrease the ability of the blood to clot; often given to patients following surgery to reduce the risk of blood clots.

Bone scan A test in which a substance is injected into a vein. If the skeletal bones are abnormal, the material accumulates in the abnormal bones, and can be detected by a special camera that takes pictures of the bones hours after the injection.

BPH See benign prostatic hyperplasia.

Brachytherapy A type of radiation therapy in which small seeds of radioactivity are placed into the prostate gland. Also called interstitial radiation therapy.

Cancer The presence of abnormal or malignant cells that have lost normal regulatory controls of growth; cancer cells may also spread to other parts of the body and grow.

Carcinoma A type of cancer that includes adenocarcinoma, or most prostate cancer.

Casodex A new antiandrogen recently approved by the FDA.

Cell The basic building blocks of all tissues and organs.

Cervical spine The vertebral bones and spinal cord where they pass through the neck.

Chemotherapy The use of specific chemicals (drugs) to eradicate cancer cells. For prostate cancer, these include estramustine, paclitaxel, vinblastine, etoposide, adriamycin, and cyclophosphamide.

Colostomy A surgical procedure in which the bowel contents empty into an opening created on the skin; usually performed when there is a blockage in the normal passageway of the bowel.

Computerized axial tomography (CAT) scan An older term for a computed tomography (CT) scan.

Congestive heart failure The inability of the heart to pump blood efficiently, causing a backup of blood and fluid in the lung area.

Core A piece of tissue which is obtained following a biopsy procedure.

Cortisone A type of medicine that contains a common type of steroid; an anti-inflammatory medicine.

Cryosurgery A surgical procedure that eliminates abnormal tissues by the use of extreme cold. In prostate gland cryosurgery, coils are placed into the gland, which freezes and eventually kills the tissue, including both cancer and normal cells.

CT scan Computed tomography, a type of radiological test in which organs can be visualized with the aid of X-rays and computers.

Cytopathologist A specialist in pathology who is able to interpret details of cellular structure.

Definitive radiation therapy The use of radiation treatments to treat and cure a patient of his or her cancerous state.

Definitive treatment The primary treatment for a disease, one that is intended to cure.

DES Diethylstilbestrol, a female hormone.

Diethylstilbestrol A female hormone used to treat men with prostate cancer by suppressing testosterone production.

Differentiated A term used to describe the normal process of cell development; applied to cancer it describes how closely the cancer does or does not resemble the organ from which it originated. The terms well differentiated, moderately differentiated, and poorly differentiated are commonly used as a way of grading cancer.

Digital rectal examination (DRE) A part of the physical examination in which the physician puts a gloved finger into the rectum and examines the prostate gland and rectum for abnormalities that can be detected by touch.

Dihydrotestosterone (DHT)   A male hormone (androgen) that influences the growth and development of both normal prostate tissue and prostate cancer.

Disseminated prostate cancer   Cancer found throughout the gland, or in the case of metastatic disease, throughout the body; opposite of focal.

Disseminated recurrence   The reappearance or return of a cancer in multiple areas of the body.

DNA   The molecule which makes up the genes and determines the inherited characteristics of the individual and the functioning of the cell, tissue, or organ.

Downstage   To lower the stage assigned to the cancer, usually following some treatment intervention.

DRE   Abbreviation for digital rectal examination.

Ejaculate   The semen; the bodily fluids (including the sperm) that are discharged through the penis during orgasm; it contains many secretions of the prostate gland.

Elevated PSA   A value of PSA which is outside and above the normal range established for the PSA test.

Embolism   The dislodging of a blood clot, allowing it to travel and lodge in another area of the body. The most serious type of embolism is a blood clot that travels to the lung (usually from the leg), causing shortness of breath and chest pain.

Emphysema   A disease characterized by progressive loss of lung function, making breathing difficult.

Epidural block   Analgesia or anesthesia produced by an injection to the area between the vertebral bones of the back.

Erectile dysfunction   A more specific term for impotence that refers to the inability to have and to maintain an erection sufficient for intercourse.

Eulexin (flutamide)   A type of antiandrogen used in the treatment of prostate cancer.

External-beam radiation therapy   A type of radiation therapy that uses an external source (called a linear accelerator) of radiation, which is aimed at the cancer.

Extracapsular   When referred to the prostate gland, the tissues surrounding the natural boundary of the prostate gland; extracapsular disease is cancer that has spread to these surrounding tissues.

Extraprostatic   Disease that has spread beyond the prostate gland.

Fecal impaction   Blockage of the bowel, usually by dried, hardened stool, usually occurring in a severely constipated patient; the blockage prevents the normal transit of fecal material along the gastrointestinal tract.

Finasteride   See Proscar.

Flutamide   See Eulexin.

Focal prostate cancer   Cancer found in one or a few small nests within the gland.

Food and Drug Administration (FDA)   The government regulatory agency that assures that new medicines and medical devices are both safe and effective prior to approval for widespread use by the public.

Frequency   The urge to urinate on a frequent basis.

Frozen section   A sample of tissue that is taken during a biopsy procedure, frozen, and then immediately examined under the microscope.

FSH   Follicle-stimulating hormone; a hormone released from the brain that controls the function of sperm production from the testis.

Gastroenterologist   A physician who specializes in the treatment of intestinal disorders; often the person who helps evaluate patients with diarrhea following treatment of prostate cancer with radiation therapy.

Gleason score   A system of identifying and grading the appearance of prostate cancer, as viewed under the microscope. Scores range from 2 to 10. Gleason was the pathologist who devised this system for assessing prostate cancer pathology.

Goserelin   See Zoladex.

Gynecomastia   Breast enlargement occurring in men.

Hesitancy   The inability to initiate a urinary stream easily; difficulty in initiating the act of urination.

Hormonal refractory disease   When referred to prostate cancer, disease that is no longer sensitive to the beneficial effects of hormonal treatments.

Hormonal therapy (for prostate cancer)   Treatments (medical or surgical) intended to reduce or eliminate the supply of male hormones to the prostate and its metastases, causing cell death and a slowing of cancer growth.

Hormonally refractory disease   A type of prostate cancer that is no longer responsive to the anticancer effects of hormonal treatments. A cancer that has become independent of growth regulation by hormones.

Hot flashes   Sweats or a hot and flushed feeling; a side effect of hormonal therapy for prostate cancer.

Hot spots   Slang term to indicate abnormal areas in the bones likely to contain cancer, as determined by bone scan.

Human-protection board   A committee of scientific and lay people, usually organized within a hospital, who oversee the use of experimental and investigational treatments, and the study of new treatments in humans.

Impotence   The inability to obtain or maintain an erection sufficient for sexual intercourse; also called erectile dysfunction.

Institutional review board   See human-protection board.

Interstitial implants   The placement of radioactive seeds into the prostate gland, usually as a treatment for prostate cancer; brachytherapy.

Interstitial radiation therapy   See brachytherapy; see interstitial implants.

Intracavernosal injection therapy   The injection of substances into the shaft of the penis to allow erection in impotent patients; a method of treating erectile dysfunction.

Investigational treatment   The use of medicines not yet formally approved by the FDA for the treatment of various disease conditions; or the use of approved medications for medical conditions when this use has not yet been approved by the FDA as an indication.

Laparoscopy   A surgical procedure in which a tube is placed into the abdomen, allowing an examination of the abdominal contents; often used to examine and biopsy lymph nodes around the prostate gland.

Latent cancer   A cancer that is detected incidentally during a patient's lifetime, but that may be an inactive cancer.

Lesion   A general term indicating any abnormality (usually found during physical examination, on radiological evaluation, or at surgery).

Leuprolide   See Lupron.

LH   Luteinizing hormone; a hormone released from the brain that controls the production of androgens from the testis.

LHRH   Luteinizing hormone-releasing hormone; a hormone released from the brain that controls the release of luteinizing hormone.

LHRH analogue   A chemical hormone similar in structure to LHRH that is used as a treatment for prostate cancer.

Linear accelerator   A type of radiation machine that delivers high-energy radiation waves to diseased areas of the body, usually in the treatment of cancer.

Localized   When used alone or with the term cancer, generally refers to cancer that is limited to a specific gland, without any distant spread; an organ-confined cancer.

Local recurrence   The reappearance or return of a cancer in a localized area, such as the prostate gland. This generally refers to an area that has previously been treated.

Lupron (leuprolide)   An LHRH analogue, used as a hormonal therapy for prostate cancer.

Lymphadenectomy   The surgical removal of lymph nodes, usually done as a staging procedure in the evaluation of patients with prostate cancer. Also called lymph-node dissection.

Lymph-node dissection   See lymphadenectomy.

Lymph nodes   Small specialized clusters of tissues that help fight infections and contain cancer cells that have moved out of a given tissue or organ.

Magnetic resonance imaging (MRI)   A test that relies on magnetic fields to visualize abnormalities in the body.

Margin   In reference to the prostate gland, the outermost surface of the gland which is removed at the time of radical prostatectomy.

Margin positive   The term used to indicate that the margin of the prostate gland, removed at surgery, contained cancer at its outermost surface.

Medical oncologist   A physician specializing in the medical treatment of cancer metastases.

Metastatic   When used alone or with the term cancer, refers to cancer which has spread throughout the body, beyond the organ or tissue in which it originated.

Micrometastases   Cancer cells outside the primary tumor, such as in the lymph nodes, which are still too small to be detected by CT or bone scan or by physical examination.

Microscopic cancer   Cancer that can be detected only with the aid of a microscope.

Moderately differentiated   A term applied to the appearance of a cancer which resembles to a moderate degree its tissue or organ of origin.

Multidisciplinary   Health-care providers from different fields who combine their expertiese and skills to provide care; a multidisciplinary approach to cancer treatment might involve physicians from different specialties, nurses, and social workers.

Multimodality   The combination of several disciplines or specialties in managing and recommending treatment for a patient with cancer. An example includes a team consisting of a surgeon, radiation therapist, and oncologist.

Myelogram   A radiological procedure that visualizes the spinal canal; it is performed by placing a substance into the spinal space that outlines the spinal cord, allowing definition of the structures of the spinal area.

Nanograms per milliliter (ng/ml)   A small quantity of a substance; one one-billionth of a gram (454 grams make 1 pound) in one one-thousandth of a liter (one liter is approximately one quart).

National Cancer Institute (NCI)   A large governmental organization that oversees the research and treatment policies for cancer; located in Bethesda, Maryland, it is part of the larger National Institutes of Health.

Neoadjuvant hormonal therapy   The use of hormonal treatment of prostate cancer prior to prostatectomy or radiation therapy.

Nerve-sparing   When referring to prostatectomy, the surgical procedure that preserves the nerves necessary for potency. Also called anatomic prostatectomy.

Neuroradiologist   A physician specializing in performing and interpreting radiological tests that evaluate the spinal cord and brain.

Neurovascular bundle   That portion of the prostate gland that contains the nerves and blood vessels necessary for the maintenance of erectile functioning and potency.

Nocturia   A condition characterized by waking from sleep with the need to urinate one or more times during the night.

Nodal   Pertaining to the lymph nodes or contained within the lymph nodes.

Nuclear medicine   The speciality concerned with the use of radioactive materials (radioisotopes) for the diagnosis and treatment of disease.

Observation Monitoring or observing a patient without performing any active interventions.

Oncologist A physician who deals with the diagnosis and treatment of cancer.

Orchiectomy The removal of the testicles, usually as a type of hormonal therapy for prostate cancer.

Organ-confined A cancer that is contained within the prostate gland without extension to the prostate capsule or beyond.

Palliative Treatments intended to relieve symptoms rather than effect a cure.

Palliative radiation therapy The use of radiation treatments to alleviate (relieve or diminish) symptoms such as pain. The treatments here are not intended to cure but rather to alleviate the symptoms of the cancer.

Pathologist A physician who specializes in the interpretation of tissues and organs as viewed under the microscope. Pathologists determine the presence or absence of cancer in tissue and organ specimens.

Pathology/pathologic findings The report of any abnormalities or signs of a disease, based on direct examination (usually by a pathologist or other physician) of tissues or organs.

Penile Of or relating to the penis.

Performance status The general state of health and functioning of an individual, evaluated using a standard numeric scale.

Perineum That portion of the body in the pelvis between the bottom of the scrotum and beginning of the anus.

Placebo A pill with no active ingredients, or a "dummy" treatment.

Poorly differentiated A term applied to the appearance of a cancer that does not resemble the organ or tissue of origin. By examining the cancer, it is difficult, if not impossible, to determine the origin of the cancer.

Positive biopsy   The presence of cancer cells in the biopsied tissue.

Postoperative   The period of time, generally thirty days, following an operation.

Preoperative   The period of time leading up to, but before an operation.

Proctitis   The inflammation of the lower rectum, generally resulting form radiation. The main symptom is diarrhea, oftentimes containing blood.

Prognosis   The prediction of how well the patient is likely to do (with or without treatment of the disease), as estimated from symptoms, pathology, and other diagnostic information.

Progression   The growth and spread of the cancer, either by direct extension or metastases.

Proscar (finasteride)   A medicine that is used for BPH; now being studied as a preventive for prostate cancer.

Prostatectomy   The surgical removal of the prostate gland.

Prostate gland   A walnut-shaped gland at the base of the bladder in males. It is involved in reproductive functioning.

Prostate-specific antigen   A substance secreted by the prostate gland, some of which passes into the bloodstream. It can be abnormally elevated in patients with prostate cancer, benign enlargement of the gland (BPH), or other conditions.

Prostatic urethra   That portion of the urethral tube that passes through the prostate gland.

Prostatitis   An infection of the prostate gland, usually by bacteria. A benign condition that can raise the PSA value.

PSA   See prostate-specific antigen.

PSA-based screening   A screening test to determine the presence of cancer in men based upon the determination of the PSA value.

PSA density   The amount of PSA (as measured in the bloodstream) divided by the volume or size of the prostate gland (as measured by ultrasound examination).

PSA velocity   The rate of change of PSA over time.

Radiation oncologist   Same as radiation therapist.

Radiation therapist   A physician specializing in using radiation to treat cancer.

Radiation therapy   A treatment designed to kill cancer cells by using high-energy waves aimed directly at the cancer-containing tissue.

Radiation treatments   The application of treatments, usually using sophisticated machines that generate radiation to treat (not diagnose) cancer.

Radical prostatectomy   A surgical procedure in which the prostate gland, seminal vesicles, and lymph nodes are removed. This is one standard procedure used for treating prostate cancer.

Radiological evaluation   A battery of tests, usually using X-ray machines and performed by a radiologist to determine the presence or absence of abnormalities in various organs throughout the body.

Radiologist   A physician who performs and interprets the results of X-ray tests, usually to diagnose various conditions; different from a radiation therapist, who treats patients with radiation.

Radiology   The branch of medicine that uses X-rays and specialized machines to diagnose various disease conditions.

Radiotherapy   Treatment with radiation.

Rectal examination   Same as DRE or digital rectal examination.

Recurrence   The reappearance or return of cancer.

Refractory (resistant)   A disease is said to be refractory when it is no longer responsive or sensitive to the treatment being given.

Regional   When used with cancer, generally refers to cancer that is no longer localized to the gland; cancer spread may be present outside the organ but is still in close proximity to it; the cancer has not yet spread to distant sites.

Remission   A condition when a cancer is under control or shrinking and responding favorably to anticancer treatment.

Residual disease   Cancer that is missed by treatment because it is undetected or proves to be more extensive than originally thought.

Restage   To reassess the anatomic areas where a cancer is located. This is usually done with the battery of tests that determined the original stage of cancer.

Risk factor   A characteristic or feature that predisposes an individual to develop a certain type of cancer or other disease.

Salvage   A term used when a secondary procedure (for example, radiation therapy or surgery) is used, following the failure of the initial treatment to control or cure the cancer.

Screening test   A test that seeks to identify the presence of an abnormal condition or disease in people who have no specific symptoms or complaints.

Scrotum   The saclike structure which contains the testes or testicles.

Seminal vesicles   Structures surrounding the prostate gland involved in storing and screening the prostate gland secretions.

Spot radiation therapy   The use of radiation therapy in limited and well-defined areas for the control of symptoms or to prevent the progression of cancer.

Stage of cancer   The level of advancement of cancer. The three general stages are localized, regional, or disseminated (or metastatic). Specific stages may be identified by number (I, II, III) or letter (A, B, C, D).

Staging tests   A series of blood tests and radiological tests that are performed to determine the extent (stage) of cancer in a patient.

Strontium   A radioactive substance that is used to help control pain from prostate cancer that has spread to the bones.

Suramin   A medicine currently being tested for usefulness in the treatment of prostate cancer.

Symptomatic   The presence of specific complaints referable to a disease process.

Syringe   A plastic cylinder with a plunger, usually attached to a needle. By inserting a needle into a tissue and pulling back on the plunger (aspiration), one can obtain cells or a piece of tissue for examination by a pathologist.

Testosterone   An androgen; a male hormone involved in the growth and development of the prostate gland and prostate cancer.

Total androgen blockade   The use of two forms of hormonal therapy (either orchiectomy and antiandrogen or LHRH analogue and antiandrogen) for the treatment of prostate cancer; also called complete androgen blockade, maximum androgen blockade, or complete hormonal therapy (CHT).

Transient   Temporary (as in a transient complication); a complication that is self-limited (does not require treatment).

Transrectal ultrasound (TRUS)   A sound wave test, using a machine inserted in the rectum, which creates a picture of the prostate gland and surrounding structures.

Transurethral   Through the urethra, usually referring to instrumentation or a surgical procedure in which an instrument is placed into and through the urethra.

Transurethral resection of the prostate (TURP)   A treatment for BPH that removes "chips" of prostate tissue through the urethra to relieve the urinary symptoms caused by benign enlargement of the gland.

TRUS   Transrectal ultrasound.

Tumor burden   A term used to describe the amount of cancer present, based upon radiological tests, surgical findings, or physical examination.

Ultrasound-guided biopsy   A needle biopsy performed by using ultrasound to visualize and target the abnormality to be sampled.

Understaging   An underestimate of the stage of the cancer, due to limitations in the sensitivity of our available diagnostic tests.

Urethral   Referring to the urethra, the tube passing from the bladder through the prostate gland to the tip of the penis in males, and the bladder to the outside in females.

Urgency   A condition indicated by the immediate necessity to urinate.

Urinary incontinence   The leakage of urine from the bladder.

Urinary retention   The inability to urinate, usually caused by a blockage to the urinary flow.

Urologist   A surgical specialist dealing with urology.

Urology   Surgery specialty dealing with diseases of the testis, bladder, kidney, and prostate gland.

Vasectomy   Surgical removal of the tube that collects secretions involved in ejaculation, generally used as a contraceptive measure in men.

Vertebral   Referring to the vertebrae, the bones that make up the back and surround the spinal cord.

Virulent   Term used to describe a cancer that behaves in an aggressive fashion by spreading or metastasizing.

Well differentiated   A term applied to the appearance of a cancer that resembles, to a great degree, its tissue or organ of origin.

X-ray   A general term used to signify the use of radiation to detect abnormalities for diagnosis, as in X-ray test.

Zoladex   An LHRH analogue, used as a hormonal therapy for prostate cancer. Also known as Goserelin.

RECOMMENDED READING AND RESOURCES

The following list of organizations, publications, and support groups represents a broad range of information services available to the patient with prostate cancer and his family. Many of the listings will be of great value to your physician and other health care providers as well since they are geared to the professional working in the prostate cancer field.

If you are aware of a resource that is not listed here, please let me know so it can be added to future editions of this book. I can be reached at the Beth Israel Hospital, 330 Brookline Avenue, Boston, MA 02215.

American Cancer Society
1599 Clifton Road N.E.
Atlanta, GA 30329-4251
1-800-ACS-2345

An excellent resource for all questions related to cancer, especially from the patient perspective. Individuals may also consult their individual state ACS societies. The Massachusetts chapter publishes a "Cancer Manual" every three to four years that is intended for physicians, but it may also be very useful for patient queries. For information on the ACS's support group for prostate cancer patients, Man to Man, call the national office or your local chapter.

*

American Foundation for Urologic Disease
300 West Pratt Street, Suite 401
Baltimore, MD 21201-2463
410-727-2908

A very helpful society providing invaluable information for patients on a wide spectrum of urologic disorders, including prostate cancer, prostate gland enlargement, and bladder and urinary problems, some of which may result from prostate cancer or its treatment. The association provides high-quality pamphlets for patients and families. They have produced a video, "Straight Talk on Prostate Health," which is available from A Vision Entertainment, 75 Rockefeller Plaza, New York, NY 10019.

*

American Urological Association (AUA)
1120 North Charles Street
Baltimore, MD 21201-5559
410-727-1100

The AUA is a major medical association, comprised predominantly of urologists, although any physician involved with the care of patients with prostatic disorders may become a member. The AUA provides invaluable service to physicians and patients alike, and distributes information geared to both a professional and lay audience. The association is also very involved with legislation efforts dealing with improvement in funding for patients afflicted with urological disorders. "AUA Today" is a newsmagazine of current concepts and the latest research news relative to many urologic disorders, with a heavy emphasis on prostate cancer.

Cancer Care, Inc.
1180 Avenue of the Americas
New York, NY 10036
212-221-3300

A superb cancer support group providing information, educational materials, and general information for patients and their families. Executive Director Diane Blum is a prominent social worker who has dedicated her professional career to helping cancer patients and their families cope with the impact of a cancer diagnosis. The group has had a long-standing interest in prostate cancer.

*

CancerNet on the Internet.
Access by getting to "Cancer Facts of the National Cancer Institute" and selecting "prostate cancer."
Internet address: http://www.ncc.go.jp

The CancerNet on the Internet is a service of the National Cancer Institute. It provides information bases, literature citations, current clinical and medical research programs, and resource listings. Information specifically directed to patients with prostate cancer is updated every two or three months. It is must reading for anyone with Internet access. Please also refer to other opportunities for new groups on the Internet relating to prostate cancer.

*

CaPCURE
1250 Fourth Street, Suite 360
Santa Monica, CA 90401
310-458-2873
Internet address: http://www.secapl.com/prostate/doc.html

This organization, founded by Michael Milken, has been extremely generous in providing much needed support for research in prostate cancer. The organization is committed to helping find a cure for prostate cancer through support of research, education, and prevention. They have the backing of prestigious scientists and clinical leaders and are quickly becoming a major force in cancer awareness. Dr. Stuart "Skip" Holden, the organization's medical director, is an articulate spokesperson who provides a balanced and knowledgeable view of critical issues facing prostate cancer research and educational efforts.

*

"From the Hill"
FMR Communications
1 Office Park West
1 Pennington–Washington Crossing Road
Pennington, NJ 08534

A periodic publication describing legislation relating to health-care issues. The publication follows legislation relating to prostate cancer screening, diagnosis, and treatment.

*

Internet access to prostate cancer information:
Access: listserv@sjuvm.stjohns.edu info
sci.med.diseases.cancer
alt.support.cancer.prostate

For those with access to the Internet, there are several very useful groups where patients discuss their individual situations, ask others for advice, and share information. It is akin to being in a discussion group where questions can be answered by both lay and professionals. Several prominent physicians and researchers dealing with prostate cancer frequently "log on" and provide reasonable answers to questions. There can be a reasonable amount of misinformation provided, but for the patient trying to get information and support from others who have gone through various treatments, or who have suffered complications, the occasional browse is strongly recommended. Another important feature is access to information. Most who write in are very anxious to share their newfound information with the universe of people on the net.

*

"The Medical Herald"
211 East 43rd Street, Suite 1600
New York, NY 10017
212-983-3525

This is an exceptional medical newspaper, aimed at the urban physician but is also useful to a lay readership, that addresses a true void in medical communication and has been on the forefront of increasing awareness of prostate cancer in African Americans and many other disorders.

*

National Cancer Institute
Office of Cancer Communications
Building 31, Room 10A24
9000 Rockville Pike
Bethesda, MD 20892
1-800-422-6237

A major government organization, associated with the National Institutes of Health, the world's largest biomedical organization, The National Cancer Institute provides a full service of up-to-date and authorative information and access to research programs nationwide. This organization is responsible for providing the information on CancerNet.

*

National Kidney and Urologic Diseases Information
    Clearinghouse
Box NKUDIC
9000 Rockville Pike
Bethesda, MD 20892
301-654-4415

This is a national organization providing useful information on a variety of disorders, with a special interest in prostate cancer and other urologic disorders. Their publications are well written and accurate.

*

"Oncology News International"
17 Prospect Street
Huntington, NY 11743

A newsletter mainly for physicians involved in the care of cancer patients. It is written in a very straightforward manner and provides valuable information for patients as well. The newsletter covers many major meetings and conferences where new information is presented months before the information appears in official medical publications.

*

Patient Advocates for Advanced Cancer Treatments (PAACT)
1143 Parmelee, NW
Grand Rapids, MI 49504
616-453-1477

A patient-advocate group that offers advice about cancer treatment options. It attempts to simplify a complicated array of choices, especially for patients with metastatic disease.

*

Pharmaceutical company support of patient educational aids and patient support:

The major pharmaceutical companies who have made a commitment to improving the care of patients with prostate cancer through new drug discovery and development have all made a major commitment to patient educational materials. These include the Schering Plough Corporation, TAP Pharmaceuticals, and Zeneca Pharmaceuticals. The educational aids include written brochures, videotapes, and audiotapes. In addition, for patients who cannot afford some of the medicines, the companies have major efforts to provide patients with means to obtain these important drugs. The companies also provide important educational aids for physicians through unrestricted grants for medical education.

Schering Plough Corporation
2000 Galloping Hill Road
Kenilworth, NJ 07033-0530
908-298-4000

TAP Pharmaceuticals
2355 Waukegan Road
Deerfield, IL 60015
1-800-809-8202

Zeneca Pharmaceuticals Group
1800 Concord Pike
Wilmington, DE 19803-2983
302-886-2231

*

"Primary Care and Cancer"
17 Prospect Street
Huntington, NY 11743
516-424-8900

"Primary Care and Cancer" is a newsletter published 10 times a year. It is predominantly intended for primary care physicians involved with cancer care, but may also be useful for patient populations. A year's subscription is $65.

*

Prostate Health Council (a division of the American Foundation for Urologic Disease, Inc.)
1-800-242-2383

This organization provides important literature for patients with prostate cancer.

*

US TOO
PO Box 7173
Oakbrook Terrace, IL
1-800-82-US-TOO
US TOO International
930 N. York Road, Suite 50
Hinsdale IL 60521-2993
708-323-1002

The US TOO organization has provided invaluable support and information for patients with prostate cancer and their families. These support groups have both patients and health professionals provide seminars and lectures on the latest developments of prostate cancer, publish newsletters, even in medical journals. The organization is dedicated to helping patients and their families gain access to information and cope with the diagnosis of prostate cancer. The literature that is published is first rate.

INDEX